CW00732067

Multisensory Rooms and Environments

also co-published with Scope (Vic.) Ltd

Sensory Stimulation
Sensory-Focused Activities for People with Physical and Multiple Disabilities
Susan Fowler
Foreword by Hilary Johnson
ISBN 978 1 84310 455 1

Anger Management
An Anger Management Training Package for Individuals with Disabilities
Hrepsime Gulbenkoglu and Nick Hagiliassis
ISBN 978 1 84310 436 0

Enhancing Self-Esteem
A Self-Esteem Training Package for Individuals with Disabilities
Nick Hagiliassis and Hrepsime Gulbenkoglu
ISBN 978 1 84310 353 0

of related interest

From Isolation to Intimacy
Making Friends without Words
Phoebe Caldwell with Jane Horwood
ISBN 978 1 84310 500 8

Quality of Life and Disability
An Approach for Community Practitioners
Ivan Brown and Roy I. Brown
Foreword by Ann Turnbull
ISBN 978 1 84310 005 8

Manual Handling in Health and Social Care
An A-Z of Law and Practice
Michael Mandelstam
ISBN 978 1 84310 041 6

Intimate and Personal Care with People with Learning Disabilities
Edited by Steven Carnaby and Paul Cambridge
ISBN 978 1 84310 130 7

Person Centred Planning and Care Management with People with Learning Disabilities
Edited by Paul Cambridge and Steven Carnaby
ISBN 978 1 84310 131 4

Planning and Support for People with Intellectual Disabilities
Issues for Case Managers and Other Professionals
Edited by Christine Bigby, Chris Fyffe and Elizabeth Ozanne
ISBN 978 1 84310 354 7

Disability and Impairment
Working with Children and Families
Peter Burke
ISBN 978 1 84310 396 7

Teaching Pupils with Severe and Complex Difficulties
Back to First Principles
Christopher Dyer
ISBN 978 1 85302 951 6

Multisensory Rooms and Environments

Controlled Sensory Experiences for People with Profound and Multiple Disabilities

Susan Fowler

Foreword by Paul Pagliano

Jessica Kingsley Publishers
London and Philadelphia

First published in 2008
by Jessica Kingsley Publishers
116 Pentonville Road
London N1 9JB, UK
and
400 Market Street, Suite 400
Philadelphia, PA 19106, USA

www.jkp.com

Copyright © Scope (Vic.) Ltd 2008
Foreword copyright © Paul Pagliano 2008
Microsoft product screen shot(s) reprinted with permission from Microsoft Corporation.

All rights reserved. No part of this publication may be reproduced in any material form (including photocopying or storing it in any medium by electronic means and whether or not transiently or incidentally to some other use of this publication) without the written permission of the copyright owner except in accordance with the provisions of the Copyright, Designs and Patents Act 1988 or under the terms of a licence issued by the Copyright Licensing Agency Ltd, Saffron House, 6–10 Kirby Street, London EC1N 8TS. Applications for the copyright owner's written permission to reproduce any part of this publication should be addressed to the publisher.

Warning: The doing of an unauthorised act in relation to a copyright work may result in both a civil claim for damages and criminal prosecution.

All pages marked ✓ may be photocopied for use with this programme, but may not be reproduced for any other purpose without the permission of the publisher.

Library of Congress Cataloging in Publication Data

Fowler, Susan, 1960-
Multisensory rooms and environments : controlled sensory experiences for people with profound and multiple disabilities / Susan Fowler. -- 1st American paperback.
p. cm.
Includes bibliographical references and index.
ISBN 978-1-84310-462-9 (pb : alk. paper) 1. People with disabilities--Rehabilitation. 2. Sensory stimulation. 3. Rooms. I. Title.
RD798.F69 2008
616.8--dc22

2007033856

British Library Cataloguing in Publication Data
A CIP catalogue record for this book is available from the British Library

ISBN 978 1 84310 462 9

Printed and bound in Great Britain by
Printwise (Haverhill) Ltd, Suffolk

This book includes a resource of ideas for sensory-focused activities. Some of the activities and equipment described in this book may not be appropriate for some individuals. It is the responsibility of the user to ensure that any activity or piece of equipment is selected and/or modified with due consideration given to the individual needs and abilities of each participant. The author cannot be held responsible for any negative consequences resulting from the use of activities in this book.

Contents

LIST OF ACTIVITIES

Foreword

What is the purpose of a multisensory room? Why have controlled sensory experiences? I have been thinking deeply about these questions for many years. After all, the normal environment is multisensory, so why have a separate dedicated space, especially when there is such a big emphasis nowadays on community inclusion for people with disabilities? As Susan Fowler points out, community inclusion and controlled sensory experiences do not have to be thought of in opposition to one another. It is not an either/or situation. Controlled sensory experiences can be used to augment community inclusion. The overriding theme of this book is the power of multisensory experiences to enrich the lives of people with profound, multiple disabilities. These experiences can occur in many different environments.

A key idea behind the use of multisensory rooms and controlled sensory experiences is for them to act as a catalyst, to provide a kick start to sensory engagement, thereby motivating the person with profound multiple disabilities to want to continue to engage in multisensory experiences in the community. Different people experience the world in different ways. For able-bodied individuals who can meaningfully engage with the normal environment, a controlled sensory experience is not necessary, although, paradoxically, much entertainment is founded on the deliberate and sustained control of sensory experience. Still, able-bodied individuals spontaneously and effortlessly become conscious of sensory experiences regardless of the type of environment they are in. The experience occurs by virtue of that person simply being in the environment and awake. If there are challenges, the individual has the wherewithal to be able to easily modify the experience to suit his or her interests and needs; for example, if it is too dark to see, use a torch.

As Susan writes, 'multisensory rooms have a place in providing opportunity and space for multisensory experiences *in addition* to those obtained throughout our regular daily activities'. I agree! Just being in the community does not necessarily result in a person being suitably enmeshed in worthwhile sensory experiences. Somewhere, along the ability continuum from able-bodied to profound multiple disability, there is a cut-off point where the environment changes from being one that can be experienced in a taken-for-granted way to one that can only be experienced if it is specifically designed to closely match the sense abilities and interests of the individual. The necessity for a controlled sensory experience arises when a person cannot or does not engage with the regular environment in meaningful ways. If it is to appeal to an individual who is already disengaged, the multisensory stimulation must be highly structured in ways that fit that person's sense abilities and interests.

All too often a person with profound multiple disability has severe problems of disengagement. Either he or she assumes a withdrawn, passive state or else he or she spends inordinate amounts of time actively involved in self-stimulation, unable or unwilling to acknowledge any form of stimulation that is not self-produced. Either way, the limited sense abilities that the individual has lie dormant. The sensory stimulation in the regular environment is insufficient to reach the threshold of meaningfulness, where some level of understanding, recognition, attending or even awareness is involved. The multisensory room can provide an environment where that threshold is crossed.

Multisensory Rooms and Environments is an important book because it provides a much needed, clear, practical, refreshing and sensible guide to staff who wish to work in this area. Susan is an occupational therapist with a wealth of experience in working with people with disabilities. She has been actively involved in the area of multisensory environments for many years and her enthusiasm for their use shines through. The book contains many well-thought-through practical activities, insightful descriptions of equipment and valuable suggestions for its effective use. I particularly liked the use of multisensory theme stories to inspire more creative use of the equipment. The book contains so many great ideas, tools and strategies to equip staff, and involve and enthral people with disabilities. I hope you enjoy and appreciate the ideas expressed in this text as much as I have.

Paul Pagliano, PhD
Associate Dean, School of Education
James Cook University
Townsville, Australia

Acknowledgements

For me, writing this book has been a very long journey. I can come up with the initial idea, but without the support of my friends and colleagues, the idea never gets past the first draft. In particular I would like to thank Ralda Bourne, who once again has managed to give me the impetus to finish this book. I would also like to thank Adrian Bone, Mandy Williams, Terry Martin, Sheridan Forster, Lee Darling, Jenny Reed, Paul Pagliano and Maureen Brewer for their input and comments.

Thanks also to the following who contributed information and ideas about equipment: Helen Dilkes, Richard Hirstwood, Flo Longhorn, Mike Ayres, Tim Swingler, Lynda Anderson, Suzanne Rizzo, Erin Smythe, Leanne Crawford, Yooralla Glenroy, Judy Denziloe, James Dean, Brigid Wright and Rod Laredo. Many an email has been exchanged as I've sought their advice on technical information and equipment ideas.

Finally I would like to thank SCOPE for supporting me with this venture and in particular Helen Larkin, Merrin McCracken and Nick Hagliassis and the team at Jessica Kingsley Publishers.

Introduction

This book is written for people with profound and multiple disabilities and those who support them. People with profound and multiple disabilities often have a combination of intellectual, physical and sensory impairments, which means that they can have difficulty interacting with their external environment and making sense of their surroundings. In particular, they may have difficulty knowing what to attend to within the multitude of sensory experiences that surround them. They may also have difficulty eliminating distractions so they can focus on a particular activity or object. Those working with other groups of people may also find this book helpful. For example, people with autism often have difficulty processing sensory information and they, too, can find the environment of daily life overwhelming. Activities that focus on the senses and the process of doing things, rather than an end product, assist in engaging and involving people with profound and multiple disabilities.

Multisensory rooms are artificially engineered environments consisting of pieces of multisensory equipment that are used to set up a specific mood in the room where activities and experiences of a sensory nature can take place. When used in a controlled way, they can help people with profound and multiple disabilities make the most of the skills they have by eliminating distractions and providing an environment that helps them interact with specific objects and people. Although the main focus in this book is on specific multisensory rooms, other artificially created environments are also mentioned.

With a philosophy and commitment to community inclusion, in the disability field it is possible to argue that it is inappropriate to write a book about multisensory rooms, which some people view as segregated settings (Whittaker 1992). However, the unique feature of the multisensory room, when designed and used correctly, is that it provides a very controllable sensory-focused environment. It can also be tailored to meet an individual's specific sensory needs and create a relaxed environment for quality personal interactions. Orr says that people may not be recognizing 'the multisensory nature of all rooms, all places' (Orr 1993, p.25). However, it can be difficult to control the amount and intensity of stimulation in the natural environment. In some circumstances, therefore, it may be more appropriate to use a controllable multisensory room. For example, some people may not benefit from going to a mainstream theatre, but a well-structured sensory-focused story run within a multisensory room may have more meaning and provide more of an opportunity for participation.

The reason for using a multisensory room is to provide a controlled, predictable and responsive environment for the person with a disability. However, chaotic and unpredictable environments are sometimes established as a consequence of the misguided design and use of a multisensory room. For example, multiple and indiscriminate pieces of equipment may be used simultaneously rather than the most suitable sensory equipment being chosen for each individual. This can have distressing consequences for some people as they struggle to make sense of an over-stimulating environment. Thousands of pounds can be spent on multisensory equipment, but little on training people to use the rooms. It is the quality of the actions of the support people setting up and using the room, not the equipment itself, that makes the room successful. It is they who ensure that the room is suitable for particular individuals, changing the environment if people become bored and under-stimulated, or removing stimuli if people become over-stimulated. Proper training can enable users to capitalize on one of the multisensory room's most unique and special features – that is, to enable sensory experiences to be delivered in a structured and controlled manner.

Little formal research has been carried out on the effectiveness of multisensory rooms and Snoezelen™ but, despite this, they have caught people's attention and proliferated in many parts of the world. Research and anecdotal evidence suggests that they help people to relax, decrease challenging behaviour, agitation and anxiety, increase interaction between people and their environment, and increase concentration (Ashby *et al.* 1995; Baker *et al.* 1997; de Bunsen 1994; Glenn, Cunningham and Shorrock 1996; Houghton *et al.* 1998; Hutchinson and Hagger 1994; Kenyon and Hong 1998; Lindsay *et al.* 1997; Long and Haig 1992; McKenzie 1995; McLarty 1993; Moffat *et al.* 1993; Morrissey 1997; Shapiro *et al.* 1997; Slevin and McClelland 1999; Terry and Hong 1998; Wilcox 1994). More research needs to be carried out in this area; however, this is not the focus of this book.

This book is written for people who are thinking of creating a multisensory room or who work in them on a regular basis. It gives people ideas as to how to set up a room and use existing equipment. It also aims to encourage people to think about multisensory experiences in a wider context – that is, not just within a multisensory room. People sometimes forget that multisensory experiences *can* and *do* take place through regular daily activities and settings. For example, multisensory experiences can be achieved from eating, drinking, showering, walking through the garden and even cleaning the house! The kitchen, bathroom, art room and beach, therefore, are all examples of multisensory environments where multisensory experiences *do* occur. However, these environments must also be set up in a structured way so that those with profound and multiple disabilities can make sense of them.

Part One of this book examines the theory and practice of behind multisensory rooms. Chapter 1 introduces the history and philosophy of such rooms, while Chapter 2 looks at many of the practicalities of planning and building a room as well as different types of designed sensory environments. Many multisensory rooms have already been built and some people are struggling to work out what to do with all the equipment once the initial excitement has worn off. To address this problem, Chapter 3 looks at using the multisensory rooms and Part Two examines multisensory equipment. After a brief introduction (Chapter 4), Chapter 5 looks at the individual pieces of equipment, presenting ideas on how they might be used. The pieces of equipment are categorized according to the sensory systems they primarily stimulate. Chapter 6, the final chapter offers some ideas for theme and story development in relation to pieces of equipment commonly found in multisensory rooms. I hope this last chapter prompts people to think of more flexible ways of using existing equipment and inspires people to introduce sensory themes and stories when working in multisensory rooms.

Note

Throughout the book, the terms 'environments' and 'spaces' are used interchangeably.

PART ONE

THEORY AND PRACTICE OF MULTISENSORY ROOMS

The Development of the Multisensory Room

This chapter looks at the history of the multisensory room, developing out of the Snoezelen™ approach and the Snoezelen™ rooms. The term 'multisensory room' is used in this book as the main emphasis is on the creation and use of a specific room that can be utilized in different ways. This chapter also looks at how the multisensory room can be used within the philosophical framework of the five service accomplishments to ensure that a quality service is provided.

The Snoezelen™ approach

Snoezelen™ rooms were originally set up as leisure facilities for people with profound and multiple disabilities. They grew out of the Snoezelen™ concept, which was developed in Holland (Hulsegge and Verheul 1987). The term 'Snoezelen™' is a contraction of two Dutch words meaning 'sniffing' and 'dozing', and is meant to convey the feeling of activity (as in sniffing) with relaxation (dozing). It is something people do rather than a specific room, so 'Snoezelen™ is an activity taking place in a dusky, attractively lit room where soft music is heard. There is an empathic appeal to the senses' (Hulsegge and Verheul 1987, p.11) where the emphasis is on just experiencing sensations, and not analysing the experiences. Hulsegge and Verheul also state that Snoezelen™ is not restricted to a particular place. Snoezelen™ is more the activity of enjoying an environment that stimulates the senses, rather than the room itself, and we can all 'snoezel'. Under this definition, Snoezelen™ can occur when having a shower, being in the park or sitting by the fire enjoying a glass of wine! The main point is that a person is enjoying the sensory aspects of the activity.

In some instances, Hulsegge and Verheul (1987) felt that everyday sensory experiences may be overwhelming for people with physical and multiple disabilities, and that there was a need for specifically developed sensory environments where sensory input could be controlled so that people could focus on one sense without being distracted. There was also a need to create an environment that people wanted to explore, because often they were not exploring their natural environment. To assist people to make the most of their sensory experiences, there was a focus on interpersonal contacts so that support people could bring equipment to those who couldn't get to it themselves and all could share the experience in an 'atmosphere of trust and relaxation' (Hutchinson and Kewin 1994, p.8).

The idea of creating specific sensory environments came from the concept of an activities tent that was set up at a centre for people with disabilities in Holland in 1978. 'The activities were meant for the lower level residents and they made use of sound, lights, balloons, hay etc.' (Hulsegge and Verheul 1987, p.24). Hulsegge and Verheul took the idea and organized a similar set-up at the De Hartenberg Institute where they worked. It began as a temporary set-up during a summer fair and developed into a large facility providing various sensory experiences.

The activity of Snoezelen™ began to take place within specifically engineered sensory environments and the term 'Snoezelen™ rooms' began to be used. However, the original concepts of Snoezelen™ were adhered to: 'The essence of the Snoezelen™ approach is to allow the individuals the time, space and opportunity to enjoy the environment at their own pace, free from the expectations of others' (Hutchinson and Kewin 1994, p.9). Snoezelen™ therefore developed into a leisure activity for people with profound multiple and physical disabilities.

Over the decades, there has been a focus on Snoezelen™ as a room rather than an activity, with Snoezelen™ meaning a specific room that has equipment to stimulate the senses. Commercial companies began to sell specific multisensory or Snoezelen™ equipment for Snoezelen™ rooms. The concept has been reinforced by the terms that some companies have used to sell their equipment, such as 'the white room' or 'the white tower' (Snoezelen™ rooms were traditionally white), and one company has trademarked the name 'Snoezelen™' for their equipment. The original idea that Snoezelen™ was an activity that could take place anywhere appears to have been lost.

Although the original Snoezelen™ facilities were developed for people with profound and multiple disabilities, they were soon being used for other populations as well and this led to rooms being used by therapists and teachers with an emphasis on education and assessment rather than just relaxation and leisure. People began to use the terms 'multisensory rooms' or 'multisensory environments' rather than Snoezelen™ rooms. For a time, there was debate as to whether people should build Snoezelen™ rooms, which had an emphasis on leisure, or multisensory rooms with a focus on education and skills training. People soon realized that these two aims were not mutually exclusive and the room could be used in many different ways depending on the equipment used and how the room was set up. The emphasis therefore shifted to building multi-purpose rooms, which could be used in different ways according to the needs of the individual.

Mike Ayres has coined the trade name Sensory Studios® to represent these multipurpose spaces:

> They [Sensory Studios®] have developed through the need for more flexible spaces which enable the users to create whatever type of environment, scene or mood they wish, either temporary or permanent. It allows appropriate interactivity by people of all cognitive and physical abilities. Sensory Studios® can be used for curriculum work, creating themed environments, specific therapy and assessment, as well as creating a relaxing or fun space to explore and experiment with. (Ayres 2001)

Pagliano (2001) also recognizes that multisensory rooms have multiple purposes and that many more people now use them. He refers to them as 'a multifunctional space': 'Multiple functions relates to clients (young infant to aged adult, profound multiple disability to dementia), facilitators (teachers, therapists, parents, caregivers, psychologists, social workers and nurses) and purpose (leisure, therapy and education)' (p.5).

Recent developments

One of the more recent developments is the mini or portable environment. Companies are selling 'sensory trolleys' (Mike Ayres), 'sensory banks' (Sensory Fun and Learning), 'sensory in a suitcase' (Kirton), 'exploring the senses kits' (ROMPA), 'sensory in a box' and 'mobile sensory rooms' (both Spacekraft). These are easy to move around and often incorporate basic equipment such as a fibre-optic spray, small mirror ball, projector, CDs and some tactile and vibrating equipment. Some companies will customize the trolleys or banks so that individuals can choose what to have in them. One company (Sensco) has developed the 'sensory corner', which incorporates a seating system and mirrors. It also has basic equipment such as a fibre-optic spray and bubble column.

The 'sensory theatre' is another expansion of the multisensory room concept, which involves a multimedia window-based package (The Sensory Company). It can be used to project pictures – for example, volcanoes – and at the same time the thunderous sounds of erupting volcanoes can be heard, while other red and yellow lights come on and off. The concept of the sensory theatre came from the idea 'to create an environment that could be controlled by every pupil and would stimulate every pupil' (Jones and Crawford 2005, p.37). A variat of Mike Ayres' studio concept, it uses completely wire-free technology (Ayres has been installing radio remote systems since 1999; Ayres 2001), so there are no switch leads to limit where a person should sit in relation to a piece of equipment. It has been used predominantly in schools.

Since its inception, the Snoezelen™ approach has evolved, not only in how it is used, but also in who uses it. Multisensory rooms are now used with adults with multiple disabilities (Ashby *et al.* 1995; Hagger and Hutchinson 1991; Hogg *et al.* 2001; Lindsay *et al.* 1997; Long and Haig 1992; Slevin and

McClelland 1999), children with disabilities (Glenn *et al.* 1996; Houghton *et al.* 1998; Mount and Cavet 1995; Pagliano 1999; Shapiro *et al.* 1997), critically ill children (White 1997), elderly people and those with dementia (Baker *et al.* 1997; Burns 2000; Hope 1999; McKenzie 1995; Moffat *et al.* 1993; Morrissey 1997; Woodrow 1998;) and for those with chronic pain (Schofield 1996, 2000; Schofield and Davies 1998; Schofield, Davies and Hutchinson 1998). They have also been used for a multitude of purposes, which include education, assessment and theme work as well as leisure and relaxation. However, it must be kept in mind that, although much of the literature supports the benefits of multisensory rooms, Martin, Gaffan and Williams (1998) concluded that it was the nature of the interactions within the environment rather than the multisensory environment itself that was of importance, while Vlaskamp *et al.*'s (2003) study suggests that the 'living unit is as good (or as bad) a place as the MSE [multisensory environment] for promoting alertness and interactions' (p.141). Finally, Cuvo, May and Post (2001) found that, when compared with an outdoor activity, the 'outdoor condition was superior' (p.183) in reducing stereotypic behaviour and increasing engagement.

The contact details for all companies mentioned in this section can be found in Appendix 1.

Philosophical framework

Multisensory rooms are one environment where sensory activities can be provided to people with profound and multiple disabilities. When thinking about activities, it is useful to think of them within a wider context to ensure that a quality service is provided. One framework to consider when thinking of quality of life issues is O'Brien's five service accomplishments (O'Brien 1989). This framework reminds us about the essential elements of a quality service delivery for people with profound and multiple disabilities, and these are now described with some discussion as to how they relate to multisensory rooms.

Respect

O'Brien emphasized that people should be respected at all times, and that our attitude is important when interacting with people who have a disability. It is how the multisensory rooms are used when working with a person that demonstrates respect for an individual.

This means that multisensory rooms should not be used indiscriminately whereby any piece of equipment is turned on and people are left isolated in an environment they did not choose. No one would like to be left in a room where physically they could not leave when they wanted to, or even turn off equipment that they disliked or found over-stimulating.

Respect also means that support people should take the time to see what people like and when they have had enough or want a change. In respecting people, we enable them to become as independent as possible, exercising choice and controlling aspects of their sensory environment.

Choice

People with profound and multiple disabilities are often not given the opportunity to make choices. However, most people are able to make choices even if they are unable to verbalize them. Time needs to be spent with people, working out how they make choices by observing their behaviours, which gives an indication of whether or not they like or dislike certain food, clothing or activities.

In terms of multisensory rooms, there are a number of ways in which choice can be offered. People have a choice whether or not they want to interact in a multisensory room. Some people may feel anxious about entering a multisensory room that is set up with dim lighting, and they may need to become used to the idea of going into this unusual sensory environment. Alternatively, they may need the environment to be set up in a different way for them to feel comfortable in it. Choice is therefore given in terms of the type of multisensory environment a person prefers, and also which type of equipment they would like to use.

Capabilities

Most people have the ability to learn or refine certain skills. It is our job to find out what motivates people and use this to help them develop their skills. This may be as simple as observing a person's reactions to certain things and how they react when they like something. If people's attempts at communication are consistently responded to, they can learn that a certain action or behaviour will bring about a certain response – that is, when they smile and look at an object they cannot reach, it will be brought to them for them to explore or use.

Within the multisensory room context, there are many skills that can be taught. These include:

- communication skills, where people are given the opportunity to interact not only with support people but also with their peers

- object engagement skills – that is, looking at the different ways people interact with different objects

- cognitive skills such as learning about cause and effect, colours, numbers and memory.

Community presence

Some people with profound and multiple disabilities may be living and working in segregated settings. With creative thinking, sensory activities within the wider community can be found that have meaning for such people. For example, there are herb gardens to visit, listening posts in music shops, perfume counters at department stores, and different textures to feel at hardware stores and haberdashery shops. A useful activity to carry out is to write down all the different things that can be experienced in the wider community, and list them under the different senses. A more comprehensive list of community sensory activities can be found in Appendix 2.

It is important to think about how multisensory rooms can be incorporated into the wider community. They could be built at mainstream schools, leisure centres, health centres or theatre complexes. These facilities could be set up to appeal to children as a play area, stressed-out adults as an environment for relaxation or massage and theatre-goers who want a multisensory experience. Multisensory environments should also be created within a person's daily life – for example, making the bathroom or kitchen a multisensory environment, or setting up a lounge room for relaxation.

Relationships

Often people with profound and multiple disabilities have restricted social networks and their main support networks include predominately paid support staff. Frequently, there is no opportunity to even interact with their peers. Part of the reason for this small social network may be due to the limited opportunity to meet new people. The other reason is that people do not always know how to communicate with a person who has complex communication needs. It is important to document how a person communicates and offer people a range of communication opportunities. If the types of objects and activities that a person likes can be determined, others can feel more confident about interacting with them, regardless of their complex communication needs, as well as giving them something to communicate about.

2

Setting up a Multisensory Room

Setting up a multisensory room isn't just about deciding you want one and looking in catalogues for equipment you might like. There is a lot of planning involved before the equipment is even chosen, and good planning helps to lead to the effective use of the room.

This chapter looks at preliminary considerations when setting up a multisensory room, which includes the rationale and issues around budget. It also looks at different types of multisensory environments that can be constructed if there is no space or desire to build a dedicated room. The final part of the chapter looks at the design and construction of the multisensory room and some general considerations in relation to equipment purchased.

Preliminary considerations

People often start thinking about pieces of equipment and room design before thinking about why they want a room and how it will be used. It is not a matter of setting up any room with any type of stimulation and bombarding a person's senses. Pagliano (2001) defined a multisensory room as 'any environment where stimulation of a multisensory nature is precisely engineered to match more closely the exceptional needs of the user' (p.34). It is imperative that, when designing and choosing equipment, people consider the individual needs of those who will be using the room as well as how the room will be used.

When thinking about design, consider the use of the multisensory room in the long term. A great room may be set up but, if it is static, people will soon become bored, so plan a flexible design.

Why have a multisensory room?

When thinking of setting up a multisensory room, it is important to begin with a series of questions rather than just seeing a room or looking in a catalogue and being impressed by the equipment that looks exciting and stimulating!

Ask yourself, 'Why do I want a multisensory room?' Some reasons for having one are as follows.

- People with profound and multiple disabilities often have sensory impairments such as reduced vision. Working in a darkened room can highlight visual objects making them easier to see. Also using fluorescent objects under UV light helps people to see things they may not see under normal lighting conditions.

- People with profound and multiple disabilities often have difficulty making sense of their environment because they do not notice objects or they have difficulty working out what to attend to. They may not have time to fully process what they are experiencing before it is gone. The multisensory room is one space where there is the opportunity to present an object again, giving people the time to notice it and decide whether or not they like something.

- By controlling the sensory input in a multisensory room, it is possible to eliminate distractions and assist people to attend to specific objects that may help them make sense of their external environment – for example, 'I felt that/saw that and I liked it.'

- Some people with profound and multiple disabilities have difficulty coping with lots of sensory stimuli at once and become anxious with the sensory overload. Sensory experience can be controlled in the sensory room, which can help reduce anxiety and increase relaxation.

- The multisensory room can provide a controllable space to assess the type of environment in which a person is most comfortable, as well as the sensory system a person appears most responsive to.

- People with profound and multiple disabilities may not find their external environment interesting to explore because they are so focused on sensations they get from their bodies (self-engagement behaviours). The multisensory room can provide novel stimuli with intense sensory input so that the environment is more interesting to explore.

- People with profound and multiple disabilities often have difficulties physically interacting with their environment. Equipment in the multisensory room can be set up so that they can interact with it easily.

- The multisensory room can provide a safe environment where people can anticipate what is going to happen next.

- The multisensory room can provide a quiet space where people have time to relax and interact with each other. This gives support people the opportunity to slow down and enjoy the company of the person with a disability, rather than focusing on a task that has to be completed. By closely observing a person's behaviour, the support person can immediately respond to any attempts at communication.

- There is also time for the support person to observe behaviours in relation to equipment in the multisensory room. They can work out whether the behaviours indicate that people are interested, disinterested or dislike equipment in the room.

- Small rooms can be built or small spaces created within a larger room, which are easier for people with profound and multiple disabilities to explore as objects, and people can be presented close to them. Some people also feel more secure exploring a smaller environment.

Remember that controlled multisensory experiences should be available to people at all times of the day and in many different environments, not just in the multisensory room.

If the decision is that a multisensory room is required, then this must be based on the needs of the people who are being supported. If so, what are their needs? Are they educational, leisure, relaxation, sensory or a mixture of these? This will have an impact on how the room is designed. Also consider if there are other ways people's needs can be met.

If someone requires sensory stimulation, what are their specific sensory needs? For example, do they need more tactile stimulation, visual, etc.? This will also determine how the room is designed and set up.

Some people may decide that it is useful to have a dedicated multisensory room, because it is impossible to create a quiet, calm space anywhere else. It is also helpful to have a space where a particular theme or story can be set up, so that it doesn't have to be packed up after each session.

How will the room be used?

This will also have implications for the design of the room. For example, how will the room be adapted to meet people's changing needs and keep it interesting? That is, how flexible is the environment?

Even if there are no specific educational goals, the room still needs to be used in a purposeful way, so how will you ensure this? This may mean that money needs to be put aside for training, so that people know how to set up the room to meet the specific needs of the people using the room. People may also need to be trained to evaluate the room, equipment or activity to ensure that it meets people's needs. Remember, it's more important *how* you use the space, not what you have in it.

Setting up the room to be interactive is crucial for the successful use of these environments. This does not necessarily mean that a person has to use a switch to operate a piece of equipment – although this is important. It also needs to be interactive socially, so that all can respond to the communication attempts of people who may be trying to share an experience or demonstrate that they like or dislike something.

Who will be involved?

When deciding to set up a multisensory room, it is important to include everyone. Not only is vital information gained from everyone on people's likes and needs, but this will also ensure that everyone will 'own' the project. In that way, it is more likely that everyone will use the multisensory room with a common agreed purpose. If people do not feel involved, they may not understand how to use the multisensory room to its fullest extent, or they may not even use the equipment at all. Worst of all, if one person is the driving force and they ultimately leave, the multisensory room may be neglected and a lot of expensive equipment that has been purchased will be wasted. If many people are involved, even if someone leaves, others can continue on, because they understand the goals and purpose of the multisensory room, and they know whom to contact if equipment needs repairing.

Health and safety issues

Think about fire safety in the design of the room. Consult with local fire officers or occupational health and safety officers to ensure the room design is safe.

Most suppliers of multisensory equipment will use fire-retardant materials. However, if people make their own equipment, ensure similar fire-retardant materials are sourced and used.

Consider people's medical conditions and whether or not different lighting effects will risk someone having a seizure or making one more severe.

Ensure that equipment is used safely by offering training in its use, and ensure that it is regularly monitored and serviced. Ensure that there are circuit breakers for the electrical equipment. Always read the warnings and safety instructions that come with any equipment.

Any equipment with a heat source – for example, the fibre-optic spray and solar projector – should be positioned where there is plenty of ventilation so that the equipment does not over-heat. Do not place heat sources on fabrics, plastic or soft play materials where there is the potential to cause a fire. Ensure electrical equipment is secured safely so that it is not accidentally knocked over.

Budget

Once people have decided that a multisensory room would be useful, they need to consider where to obtain the money to convert a space and to buy equipment. There may be a budget available but, more usually, someone or a group of people will need to be responsible to apply for a grant or organize fundraising. People can often fundraise for initial equipment because it is tangible and novel, but it is more difficult to gain funds for maintenance.

Large amounts of money do not need to be spent to set up a multisensory room, and interesting mini-multisensory environments can be created with a small budget. People are often seduced by glossy catalogues and think that they need to purchase lots of expensive high-tech equipment.

If there is a restricted budget, think about low-tech equipment that can be made easily – for example, make textured mats, create a vibrating bed by placing a vibrating snake underneath one corner of a lilo, or purchase a vibrating mat. Mini-environments can also be created by attaching strips of fluorescent kite material (ripstop nylon) around a hoop (as in Figure 2.1), suspending it from the ceiling, seating a person under it and attaching a fan to a power box. The person can then operate the fan to set the streamers moving around them. To make the experience more visual, direct a spotlight or UV light onto the streamers.

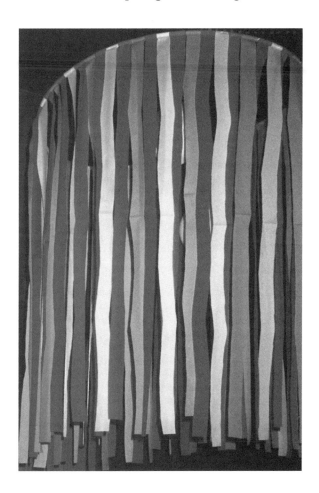

Figure 2.1 Fluorescent hoop

When thinking about money needed for a multisensory room, many people just focus on the equipment. However, there are additional costs, especially if the intention is to set up a dedicated room. Some of these 'hidden' costs include:

- electrical wiring (which can be very expensive)
- ventilation
- room conversion (such as knocking down walls)
- storage

- painting

- flooring

- maintenance, cleaning and management overheads

- a person's time to research multisensory rooms, order, chase up or make equipment

- training in the use of the multisensory room

- a person's time to show other interested people around the multisensory room

- new equipment, maintaining a replacement fund for old equipment, repairs to equipment and funding for spare parts such as globes or light bulbs.

Multisensory rooms should be fluid so it doesn't matter if the budget does not cover all the expensive pieces of equipment straightaway. However, if planning to buy a big piece of equipment in the future, this needs to be incorporated into the initial design. This may mean planning for an extra power socket and thinking about where the equipment will be placed so that there is room for it in the future.

If purchasing equipment from specialist companies, some will include installation costs in their quote. If they do not, be aware that there will be an additional cost in terms of money or time. Some companies will also carry out the whole project, converting the room and installing the equipment. This may not be the option required, because any one company may not provide all the equipment needed. Some people choose to buy some pieces of equipment from one company, other pieces from another company, and make and source other equipment themselves.

Designed multisensory environments

Broadly, there are two types of multisensory environments – natural and designed. Natural environments are ones that have not been specifically created to provide multisensory input, but provide multisensory experience as part of everyday life – for example, at the market or on the beach.

We live in a multisensory world but some people require specifically designed multisensory environments because they can become overwhelmed by the multitude and intensity of sensory stimuli in the natural world. The designed environment can also be created with the specific needs of users in mind and provide people with the opportunity to have control over their environment, something they may have difficulty doing in their natural environment.

Purpose-built multisensory rooms can provide structured sensory environments; however, it is not necessary to set up a specific multisensory room to provide controlled multisensory experiences. Thus, a relaxing ambience can be created in a person's own lounge room by dimming the lights, listening to relaxing music and having a massage with relaxing aromatic oils.

Multisensory rooms are only one type of purpose-built multisensory environment (MSE). However, the term 'MSE' can be used in a very broad sense and can mean anything that's designed to provide multisensory stimulation in a person's external surroundings. Thus, an activity arch (as in Figure 2.2) set up around a person's wheelchair that may have bells, textures or a mini mirror ball hanging from it can be just as much an MSE as a dedicated room with a multitude of multisensory equipment.

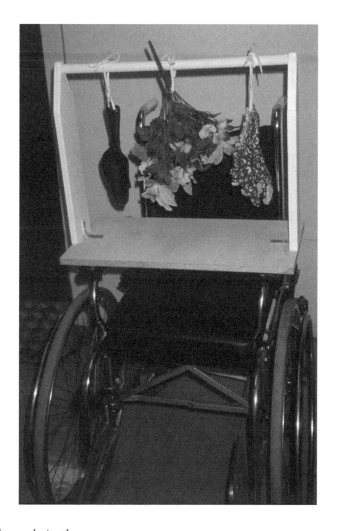

Figure 2.2 Activity arch example with a gardening theme

Sensory banks are a useful way of storing sensory equipment so that it is available to use in various types of multisensory environments. Appendix 3 gives more information on sensory banks and the types of materials that can be stored in them.

Other examples of designed MSEs are as follows.

Dark room

Dark rooms are rooms that have normal light excluded and are traditionally painted black. This is to eliminate any visual distractions so that torches and UV lights can be used to highlight particular objects. They are used mainly as an environment to stimulate and enhance visual skills.

Dark rooms have often tended to be small spaces and, when painted black, they can feel very claustrophobic and threatening for some people. It is not necessary to paint a dark room black: light just needs to be eliminated so that, when objects are highlighted with spotlights, torches or UV lights, they visually stand out from the background environment. Another alternative is to use a large box painted black as a mini dark room.

It is important to ensure that the dark room does not become cluttered with objects. The objective of a dark room is to screen out excessive visual stimuli and thus reduce distractions so that a person can concentrate on a particular visual object or activity. It is therefore important to have storage areas for the dark room so that unnecessary equipment can be put away during an activity.

Sound rooms

Sound rooms are specialized sensory environments concentrating on using sound as the main sensory modality. Effective sound environments can be created based on using musical instruments and the Soundbeam (see Figure 2.3). The Soundbeam is a piece of equipment with an ultrasonic sensor that is attached to a keyboard or sound module.

The Soundbeam creates a virtual keyboard or musical instrument in space that can be 'played' in response to people's movements. As people move through

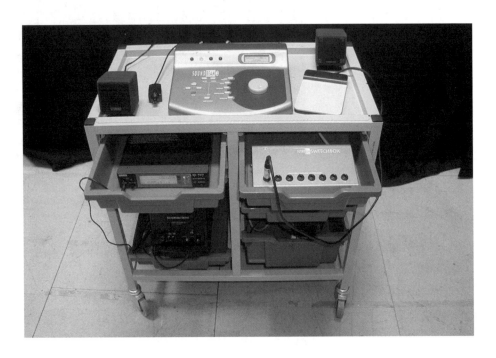

Figure 2.3 The Soundbeam

this invisible beam, it triggers the notes or sounds of the keyboard or sound module. This means that people can create interesting sounds even with the smallest movements.

The Soundbeam can also be used in conjunction with other equipment so that people can explore sound and movement.

If a sound box (as in Figures 2.4 and 2.5) is attached to the Soundbeam, people can feel the vibrations from the Soundbeam through their feet or body, depending on whether they are sitting or lying down. Vibroacoustic beanbags (see Figure 2.6) or body pillows are also available, whereby people can recline in a beanbag and also feel the vibrations from music or the Soundbeam.

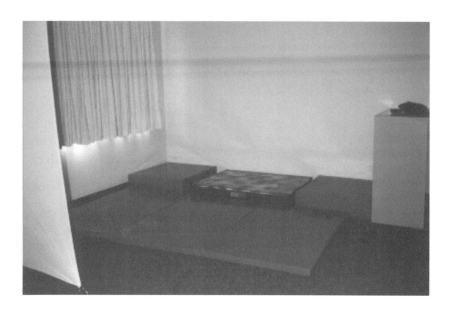

Figure 2.4 Soundbeam box

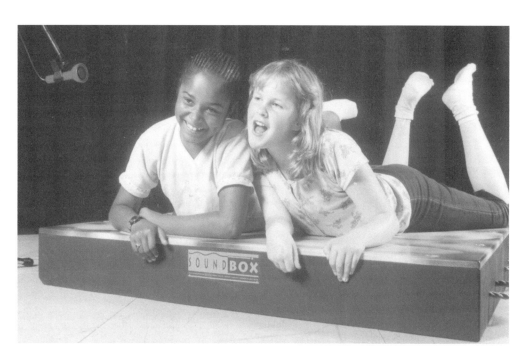

Figure 2.5 Sound box

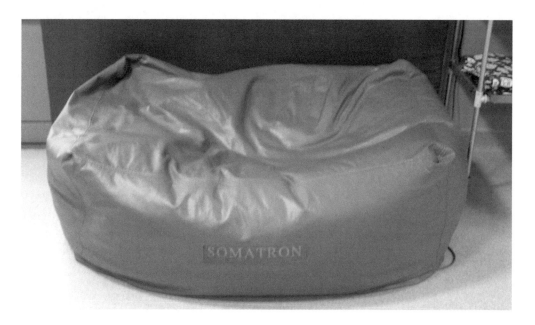

Figure 2.6 Vibroacoustic beanbag

Ceiling grids (as in Figure 2.7), first introduced into rooms and studios by Mike Ayres as long ago as 1989, are frames suspended from the ceiling, and can be used as structures from which to suspend wind chimes (metal or bamboo) or other equipment. These chimes can be set in motion by using a fan. Storage cupboards are necessary to house other sounding instruments such as a Mexican rain stick, maracas, claves and egg shakers.

To introduce visual stimulation, Helen Dilkes, a soundscape researcher in Victoria, Australia, has created a projection curtain or shadow screen using a piece of white Lycra® (as in Figure 2.8). The Lycra® can be suspended from the ceiling grid and fixed to the floor using sandbags. On one side of this screen is a spotlight so that, when people move in the Soundbeam, their shadows are seen on the other side of the screen (as in Figure 2.9).

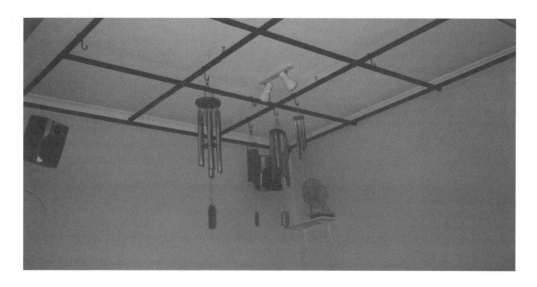

Figure 2.7 Ceiling grid

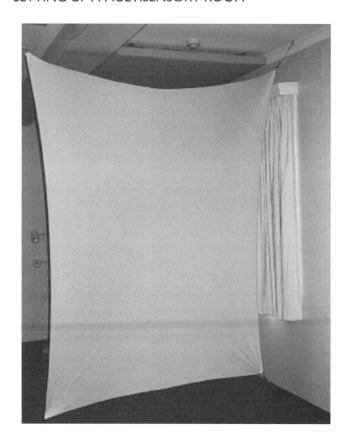

Figure 2.8 Soundbeam screen

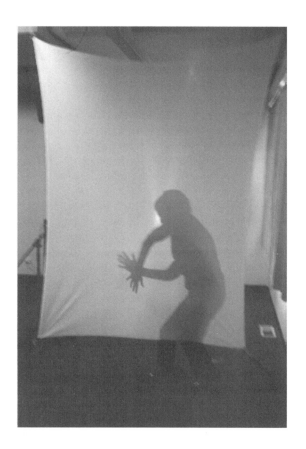

Figure 2.9 Shadow

Sensory tent

This is one way to create a mini sensory environment, which some people find more secure than being in a big open room. Three-sided beach tents, which are used to provide shade and wind protection, can easily be converted into a mini-MSE. Hoops, shoelaces or elastic can be sewn or velcroed onto the tent so that equipment can be suspended (as in Figure 2.10). Textured rugs and other textured items can be provided for people to explore. Some tents are darkened for visual activities by draping a cloth over the tent. Mini mirror balls can be fixed to the inside of the tent and a table lamp can be angled to shine onto the mirror balls. Some tents are set up to be interactive whereby people can turn on a fan to set bells chiming or streamers moving. People can also turn on a light themselves by using a touch lamp or a switch linked to a lamp through a power box. A power box (see p.50) can be used with a piece of equipment that is powered by mains electricity. It has a socket for a switch so that people who are unable to use the switch on the electrical device can use an external switch, which they find easier to operate – for example, by rolling on a mat switch, using their chin with a small button switch, or reaching out to press a large round switch.

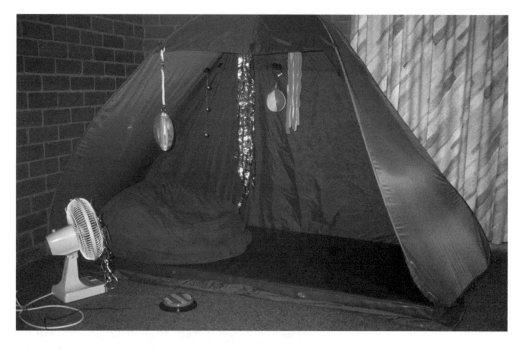

Figure 2.10 Sensory tent with fan

Theme corner

MSEs do not have to be set up in a dedicated room: a corner of a room can be set up as an MSE. An effective approach to set up a mini-environment is to base it on a theme – for example, related to seasons, places people have visited, or relevant to people's interests. One idea is to set up a fish theme, where silver streamers and blue cellophane represent the sea. Large fish kites can be hung in front of the cellophane. To make the environment interactive, a fan attached to a power box can be used to make the streamers and fish move (see Figure 2.11). Bowls of sand, water, sea sponges, dried seaweed, dried starfish and shells can also be provided to allow opportunities to experience a variety of textures.

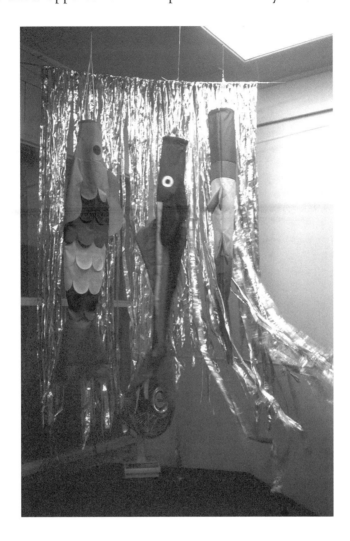

Figure 2.11 Fish corner

Computers

Computers can be used to create multisensory environments. Packages such as Microsoft's PowerPoint can easily be utilized to make slide shows incorporating photographs and recorded sound. For example, a group project might be to take photographs of different animals or transport and then record in the corresponding sounds.

Computers can also provide tactile experiences in terms of vibration as interactive cushions are now available (see Figure 2.12).

These are plugged into the computer and respond to the different sounds made in computer games and music. Other ways to incorporate tactile experiences are to use tactile switches (as in Figure 2.13) and overlays, such as bubble wrap, fur and corrugated card, on expanded keyboards.

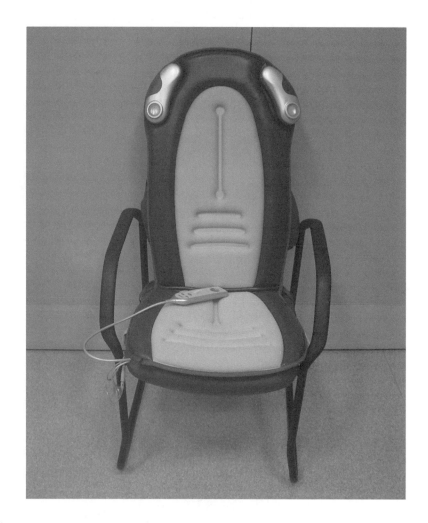

Figure 2.12 Interactive cushion

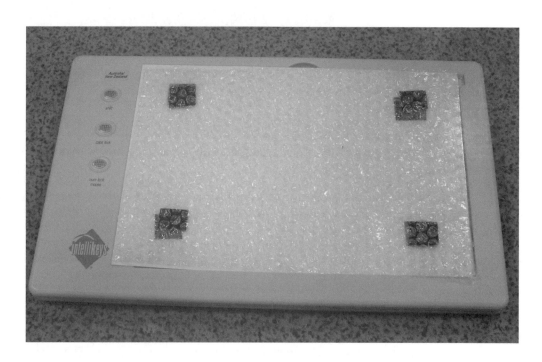

Figure 2.13 Tactile switch made with bubble wrap

Sensory gardens

Gardens are natural multisensory environments; however, sensory gardens are planned to maximize the sensory components of a garden. To plan a sensory garden, first think about the different senses and how these can be incorporated into a garden. Some ideas are now listed under the different senses.

TOUCH

There are many types of plants with different foliage as well as the bark and nuts that can be felt on trees. Gardens can be planned with different surfaces to walk on and sensory walls (as in Figure 2.14) can be made using plumbing materials – for example, plastic grilles and piping. Consider, also, different sculptures and mosaics that can be incorporated into the garden to provide further diversity of tactile surfaces.

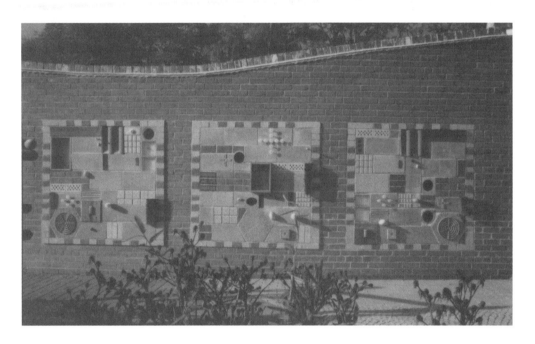

Figure 2.14 Tactile wall

SEEING

There are so many plants that produce a variety of colour in the garden. Think about putting clusters of the same colour together to make it easier for people with vision impairment to see. Particular plants can also be used to define areas such as paths. Also remember to install plants that attract birds and butterflies, in order to provide further visual stimulation.

HEARING

A variety of path surfaces with different textures can provide auditory stimulation as a person walks or a wheelchair is propelled over them. Again, trees that attract birds will also provide auditory stimulation in terms of bird calls and bird songs. There are many different wind chimes that can be purchased or made that produce various sounds – for example, wind chimes made from bamboo or kitchen utensils (see Figure 2.15).

Think about having a water feature – not only is it soothing to listen to, but it is visually relaxing.

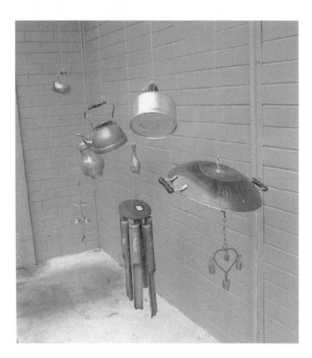 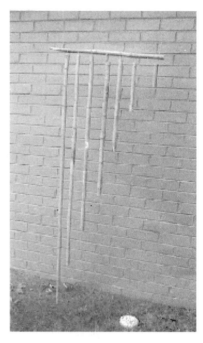

Figure 2.15 Wind chimes

Large gardens can incorporate a 'sound sculpture'. One such sculpture was completed as a group project where pipes of various lengths were cut and later strung out in the garden. The length of the pipe was determined by the length of the different parts of people's bodies – for example, length of arm or leg, length from shoulder to elbow. People then listened to the sounds that their individual pieces of piping made, before it was all pieced together as one structure.

SMELL

When planning a sensory garden, think about the different scents from the flowers and herbs. Freshly mown grass and compost also have very strong smells.

TASTE

There are many plants that can easily be grown and later used for cooking – for example, vegetables, fruits and herbs.

For more information on sensory gardens, refer to the following publications by the Horticultural Therapy Association of Victoria, *An Introduction to Raised Garden Beds* (1996), *Sensory Gardens for Horticultural Therapy Programs* (1997), and the excellent book by Monty Don, *The Sensuous Garden* (2001).

The following websites provide information on UK approaches to sensory gardens:

- www.ltl.org.uk
- www.noahsarkgardens.co.uk
- www.nurseryworld.co.uk
- www.rhs.org.uk
- www.rnib.org.uk
- www.sense.org.uk
- www.sensorytrust.org.uk

The current emphasis in the UK is for inclusive gardens.

Design and construction of a multisensory room

Structural design

EXISTING SPACE

Decide if there is enough space to dedicate an entire room as a multisensory room, or whether a corner of an existing activity room, classroom, lounge area or bedroom will be used instead. If there are a number of rooms that can be used, decide which would be the most useful in terms of size, access and ease of conversion. Consider making a sketch of the existing place, putting in doors, windows and other immovable pieces of furniture. This gives a clear picture of the space available to install equipment. Remember to include storage and access to/from the room and to/from the equipment. If there is already some equipment available for the multisensory room, sketch it into the plan as well.

Very few people have the luxury of building a sensory room from scratch. More usually, a space has to be found within an existing building. When looking at existing space, consider the following.

Overall dimensions

What are the dimensions of the space that is being considered for a multisensory room? Will it be large or small? Small spaces are useful for carrying out assessments or one-to-one skills-based training. Smaller rooms also prevent large groups of people being left in a room. However, a larger space is necessary if it is to be used as a multisensory theatre.

If undertaking assessments, it is more useful to work on a one-to-one basis so that even small behavioural changes can be observed. Also, if teaching more than one person at a time to use a switch, it can be confusing. How can a person learn cause and effect if an effect is occurring because another person used their switch but they didn't?

Another option is to think about how to divide up the space. This has a number of advantages. If the room is too large, the feeling of security can be lost and it can be difficult to establish rapport with a person. If the space is divided up, people can carry out different activities in different sections without interfering with each other. On other occasions, the space can be opened up for use as a multisensory theatre.

One way of dividing up the space is to use curtains of different material. These can be pulled across as needed. Think about creating small spaces over particular pieces of equipment – for example, draping a mosquito net over a leaf chair or hanging lace curtains over a vibrating bed.

Walls, windows and doors

When looking at the existing space, remember to draw a plan, putting in the doors and windows. How will these impact on the design? There may be a need for a large vibrating bed, but not enough wall space because of doorways. There may also be a need for a large tactile wall, but no uninterrupted space because of windows. Is it feasible to have a tactile wall that fits under the windows? This may be especially useful if the people using the wall are not ambulant and will be using the wall lying down. Another idea is to have a window unit built with coloured Perspex™ so that, when the sun shines through the Perspex™, it casts multicoloured dots on the floor.

Built-in furnishings and anything else immovable

Anything that cannot be moved out of the room will have an impact on the design. With creative thinking, these features can be incorporated into the design. For example, Toowoomba West Special School in Queensland, Australia, converted a storeroom into a multisensory room. The storeroom (see Figure 2.16) was transformed into a forest glade and the ugly hot-water system that could not be moved was converted into an attractive cottage (see Figure 2.17).

CEILING GRIDS (SEE FIGURE 2.7 ON PAGE 34)

Ceiling grids are useful to install because they create flexibility in the design of the room. They are frames suspended from the ceiling in a grid pattern so that there are a number of points from which items may be suspended. They can be used to suspend curtains of different textures or to hang different pieces of equipment. In this way, the atmosphere of the room can easily be changed or different themes can be incorporated. If there is no money to install a ceiling grid, a rod or line can be used to hang pieces of fabric or different pieces of equipment, but the hanging area will not be extensive. Hanging a sheet of white fabric can create a projection screen. Scrunching up a ball of tulle, lace or

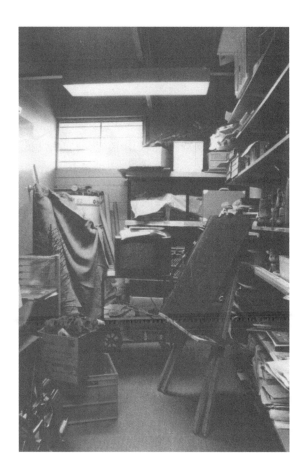

Figure 2.16 Storeroom

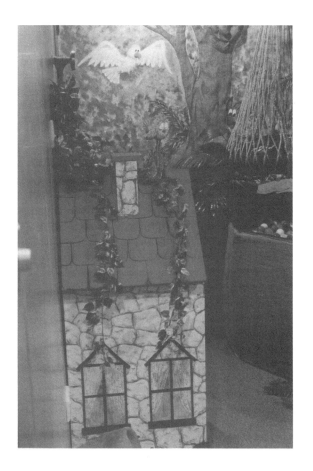

Figure 2.17 Hot-water system as cottage

survival blankets, suspending white streamers or using a white umbrella can also create projection surfaces.

HOISTS

When working with people with physical disabilities, hoists are a necessity. Where possible, install a ceiling hoist, especially if the room is small, because this gives more room to manoeuvre. If installing an electric ceiling hoist, have the ceiling checked to ensure that it is safe to carry the hoist. Also remember to install a power socket up near the ceiling so that the hoist can be powered and recharged. If portable hoists are the only possibility, remember to incorporate them in the design. For some equipment such as a ball pool or vibrating bed, be sure that the legs of the hoist can fit underneath.

VENTILATION AND HEATING

Often multisensory rooms will become quite warm, especially if they are small and the windows are blocked. Think about how the room will be ventilated, especially in summer. Conversely, in winter, think about how the room can be kept warm. Concentration is difficult if the temperature of the room is not correct, and it is very difficult to relax if it is too cold.

STORAGE AREAS

One common mistake made when setting up a multisensory room is that too much equipment is installed so the area becomes cluttered and visually very busy. This is especially a problem for people with vision impairment because some are not able to make sense of their visual environment. To avoid this problem, it is better to install a few large pieces of equipment and keep the rest stored away in cupboards or behind curtains until they are required.

WINDOW COVERINGS

Many existing spaces have windows that will need to be darkened if light effects are to be used. Windows can be painted black, but this is a relatively permanent effect and not very useful in a multi-purpose space. The same can be said for putting board over the windows. This is suitable if the room is not a multi-purpose space and a permanently dark room is required. However, this is only an option when there is another source of ventilation. Curtains or blinds may be an option but they can let in some light. Remember to think about using blackout backing on the curtains.

FLOORING – MATS, TYPE, COLOUR

A traditional Snoezelen™ or white room will often have wall-to-wall mats on the floor. This may be comfortable for some people, but for others it provides a very unstable surface upon which to walk, making it difficult for them to move around independently. Also, people in wheelchairs will have difficulty accessing the room. A better solution may be to have pathways between mats where people can move on a stable firm surface from one area to another. Different floor surfaces also help people to differentiate between the different parts of the room.

If using carpet in the room, remember to look for a low-pile carpet that is firm to walk on and easy to push wheelchairs over. Also look at how easy it is to clean that type of carpet. Again, like the walls, go for plain colours. If the floor is highly patterned, it will detract from the other features in the environment. Some people advocate grey carpets, because they are a neutral colour on which to build. Also remember that using different coloured carpet tiles as well as different textures can delineate areas. Do not be tempted to delineate an area using a rug or carpet because people can trip over loose mats.

Another way of marking out an area is to use different coloured soft play mats. Some people have used mats that are white on one side and coloured on the other. Another option is to have white on one side and black on the other as the black will show up some of the pieces of equipment more effectively – for example, the fibre-optic spray and UV objects.

SEATING

Traditionally, Snoezelen™ white rooms have used white mats and beanbags for seating. However, some people, especially older people, find it threatening and/or difficult to sit on the floor. Other comfortable and supportive chairs are therefore needed in a multisensory room. A person's own lounge room can be made into a simple relaxing multisensory environment using the usual lounge chairs. Just add some soothing music, relaxing essential oils, soft tactile covers for the chairs or chair arms (e.g. lambswool) and maybe a visual item as a focus of attention.

Leaf chairs (see Figure 2.18) have become very popular in multisensory rooms. These are seats that give support and provide movement stimulation. They can be suspended from the ceiling, or from a stand so that the leaf chair is freestanding. This is an option if the ceilings cannot support the weight of the chair, but they do take up a lot of room. When using a leaf chair, think about how a person will be secure in it – for example, do they require a safety strap? Transferring in and out of a leaf chair can be a concern because it is suspended and will therefore move freely. Plan how it will be anchored to ensure that people transfer safely.

Another popular seat is the vibroacoustic beanbag (see Figure 2.6 on p.34), which is attached to a stereo system and has speakers inside. When music is played, people can feel the beat of the music through the beanbag. Deep bass beats are most effectively felt.

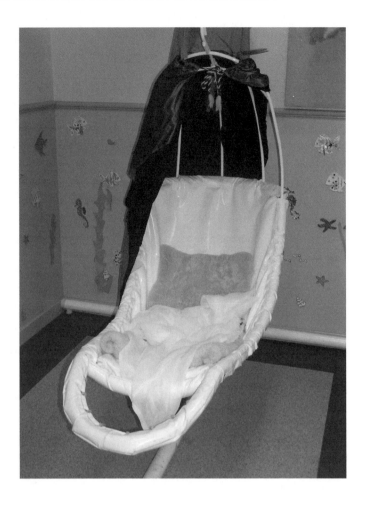

Figure 2.18 Leaf chair

COLOUR OF THE ROOM

If the Snoezelen™ philosophy is followed, rooms generally will be painted white. The main reason for this is that there are a lot of visual effects in this type of room and they show up better when projected onto a white background.

The problem with a totally white room is that it can appear clinical. However, proponents of white rooms argue that the room will hardly ever be 'white' as such, because some light effects will always be on. Of more importance is the impact the room has on people with a visual impairment. It can be very difficult for people to make their way around the room and make sense of what is happening if there are very few visual cues. How do they differentiate between the walls and floors if they are both white? How do they find the door if the walls, door and doorframe are white? How easy is it to differentiate between the walls and the door? If the room is white, think about highlighting important features, such as doorways, with different colours.

One final problem with white rooms, especially if many of the mats and other soft play pieces of equipment are white, is keeping the whole room clean. The multisensory room may look good for a few months (or in some cases days or weeks!), but the walls and white furnishings can soon look grubby and give the whole room a shabby appearance.

Another popular colour for use in a multisensory room is black, especially where UV equipment is used. This can be claustrophobic for some people, especially if the room is small to start with. Some people also find it threatening to go into a small black room.

More usually these days, a UV area will be set up within a room rather than be a space on its own. Some people have created dark and white areas within the same room, but have divided the space using thick fabric with white on one side and black on the other. Some rooms have been painted ivory and dark blue to get away from the clinical look and the overpowering effect of a completely black room.

Often multisensory rooms will be set up in multi-purpose areas or in a home lounge room, where it is not practical to paint the walls white or black. Any plain, light colour upon which to project light effects is acceptable. More important than the colour of the walls is the ability to darken the room to show up light effects, especially if using UV equipment, and also having a plain background on which to project light.

ACOUSTICS

Some rooms tend to be very noisy, especially if they have linoleum floors and few soft furnishings. Some equipment, such as ball pools that have a ball dumper, can be quite noisy. The noise from these types of equipment can interfere with other activities in neighbouring rooms. If this is the case, think about how the noise level can be reduced. Installing carpets, curtains, mats and soft furnishings can deaden the noise. Acoustic panels, which can be hung or attached to the ceiling (see Figure 2.19), may need to be installed. However, be aware that these acoustic panels can be costly.

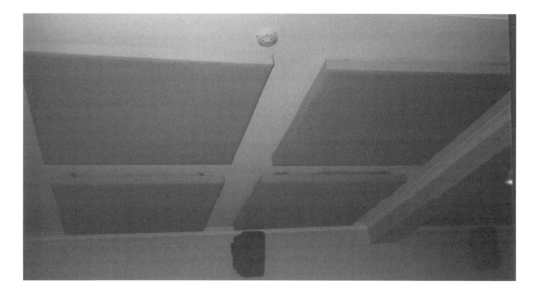

Figure 2.19 Acoustic ceiling panels

Electrical design

LIGHTING

Rooms often have bright fluorescent tubes for lights. However, this type of lighting may be too harsh to use in a multisensory room. It may be necessary to have it for cleaning purposes or to set up the room, but it is not a particularly relaxing type of light. If the room has been set up so that someone can relax, turning on bright, harsh lights when they leave could negate the relaxing effects that were produced. Using a dimmer switch can gradually increase lighting.

It is also important to have lighting that can be varied, because some people may need quite bright light initially to feel safe enough to venture into the room. Some people love to walk into a multisensory room that is already set up with subdued lighting and interesting visual effects. However, for others, this is too threatening and they need to come into a normally lit room at first; then the lighting can gradually be turned down.

Spotlights are useful because they can create different effects in the room, or highlight certain features of the room. Remember different coloured spotlights can be purchased. The different coloured lights can be used to create interesting visual effects when shone onto different materials – for example, lace (see Figure 2.20).

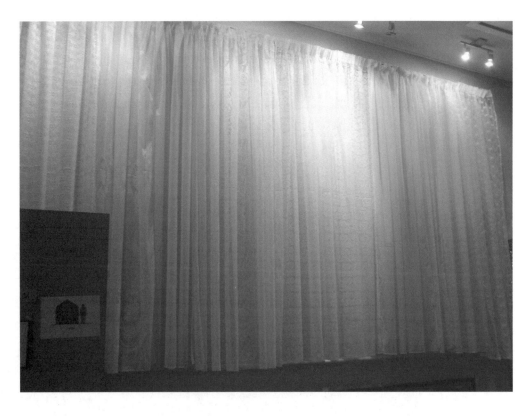

Figure 2.20 Coloured lights on lace

A bright light can be used to assess whether or not people can see light. If the room is in darkness and the spotlight suddenly comes on, some people will become still if they have been moving their head around and others will look for the light source, demonstrating that they are responding to light.

To make the room interactive, think about connecting the spotlights to a switching system so that people can change the atmosphere in the room. Spotlights can be used to highlight people or objects in the room. For example, multisensory rooms often have mirror balls and spotlights, and people can create an immediate interesting visual effect by turning on a spotlight that is projected onto a mirror ball. At one moment, the room may be dimly lit but, once they use a switch, the room is filled with coloured spots of light that move if the mirror ball is rotating. When installing the mirror ball, think about the effects required because these will determine where it is positioned. Refer to the equipment section of this chapter for more information.

POWER SUPPLY

There are never too many electrical sockets! Much of the equipment used in multisensory rooms is operated through mains power and there is nothing worse than having extension leads and double plugs all over the room. Not only is it unsightly but it is potentially unsafe. It is also important to have an approved safety switch installed to ensure safety when using the electrical equipment.

Think about the position of the sockets. Remember that some equipment such as mirror balls are often mounted on or near the ceiling, and those that rotate will need a power socket. Some equipment has a black power supply adaptor that takes up more room than an ordinary plug, so allow the space for this. Be sure to seek professional advice from a licensed electrician when setting up a multisensory room.

CONTROL SYSTEMS (SWITCHING)

In the past, traditional Snoezelen™ rooms were passive in terms of controllability of equipment. These days, integrated switching systems are often installed so that leads can be safely hidden behind walls. It is vital that the rooms are interactive because one of the main benefits of multisensory rooms is that people have control over the equipment. This helps them to learn concepts such as cause and effect, which show them that they can have an effect on their environment. This can enhance people's motivation to explore and can assist in improving self-esteem.

Companies providing multisensory equipment provide control systems or built-in switching systems. However, be very clear about how the room is to operate because some electricians who do not have experience with multisensory rooms may have difficulty setting up the room in the way you wish. Also ensure that whoever does the wiring clearly labels the switches so that everyone knows how to turn on all the equipment.

Integrated switching systems can be expensive, and one of the cheapest ways to make individual pieces of equipment interactive is to use a power box or power link (see Figure 2.21). Refer to the manufacturers' instructions before using the power boxes in order to ensure that the particular model being used can cope with the equipment.

The power box has three modes of use:

1.   Momentary/direct – the equipment will only stay on while people have the switch held down.

2.   Timed – the equipment will stay on for a predetermined time before stopping. The length of time the piece of equipment works can be preset. People need to use the switch again to turn the equipment back on.

3.   Latched – the switch is used to turn the equipment on, then used again to turn it off.

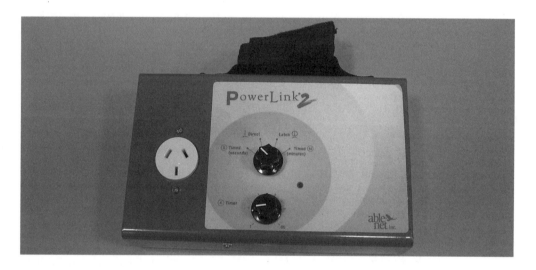

Figure 2.21 A power box

The timing option is useful for encouraging people to use switches. If the switch is linked up to a piece of equipment they really enjoy, they will be more motivated to use the switch to turn it back on. If a piece of equipment is on all the time, not only will they have no reason to use a switch, but the sensory effect of that piece of equipment can wear off. People become accustomed to it and don't notice it any more. If the equipment suddenly goes off, there is a change in the environment that can arouse people.

When considering the type of switching system to install, remember to put aside money to purchase different types of switches. This will ensure that people can turn on equipment in different ways, using different parts of their body as well as developing fine motor skills. Types of switches can include big switches, small button switches, lever switches, string pull switches, grip, wand and finger isolation switches, sound switches (used by people vocalizing to operate a piece of equipment) and mat switches. Mat switches are useful to encourage people to move and explore the space around them. By placing the mat switch near the person lying on the floor, they can operate the equipment by rolling onto the mat. Tactile switches can be bought commercially, which have different textures such as raised bumps of plastic or koosh ball switches. Textured switches can also be made by using Velcro® to put different textures onto a basic switch or making covers for mat switches (see Figure 2.22).

Radio-controlled switches have been available since 1999 when Mike Ayres

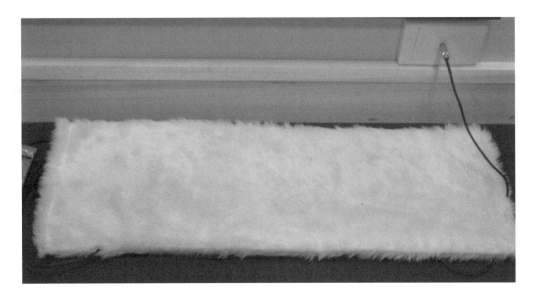

Figure 2.22 Tactile cover for switches

first used them. These eliminate the need for leads to trail from the switches to the equipment. Check that the radio-controlled switches have timing components, so the equipment can be turned on immediately or left to run for a period of time before people have to use the switch again.

Switches can also be used with battery-operated equipment through the use of a battery interrupter (see Figure 2.23). This consists of a lead with a metal plate which inserts in the battery compartment at one end and a switch socket at the other.

Although it is important to have a switch interactive environment, for some people, such as those with autism, it may be better to position the switches so that they are not accessible. People with autism often have difficulties with social interaction, and a sensory environment that they can operate without the need to communicate with anyone may encourage them to withdraw further into their own private worlds. In this instance, it may be better to teach them to use a person as a switch rather than an object switch. So, put the switches up out of the way so that they have to communicate with a support person to get the switch or turn on the equipment.

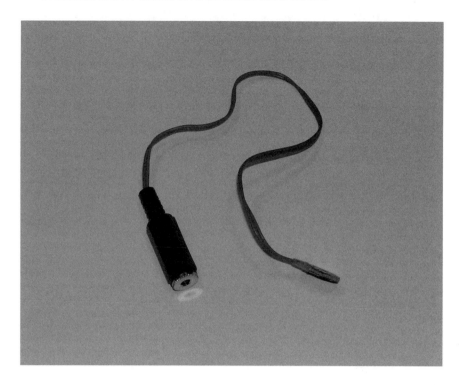

Figure 2.23 Battery interrupter

Equipment

It is important to think about buying equipment that will provide an interactive and versatile sensory room, which is flexible so that it can meet the needs of everyone and the changing needs of one person. To help with decisions about which equipment to buy, look at catalogues, visit other multisensory rooms and talk to people who are using them. Ask them a number of questions: what works, what doesn't, what they would do differently next time, how they are using their multisensory rooms and the pieces of equipment in them, and which pieces of equipment they find most useful and why.

When drawing up a list of equipment, there are a number of considerations as follows.

Flexibility and multiple purposes

Think about the different uses for each piece of equipment, especially if it is expensive. Equipment items need to be flexible and multi-purpose; otherwise, people will soon become bored with them.

Cheap versus expensive equipment

Do not think that all the sensory equipment needs to come from companies selling multisensory equipment. These pieces of equipment may be exciting for some, but not necessarily for a person who has a disability. Remember when working with people with profound physical and multiple disabilities that they may not be interested in all the equipment like the solar projector that produces stunning visual effects: they may be more interested in something that vibrates, such as a vibrating mat.

Equipment purchased for multisensory rooms tends to be very expensive, especially if the equipment is imported from overseas, and where manufacture is small scale and labour intensive. Remember that sometimes cheaper pieces of sensory equipment can be bought from normal commercial outlets. Also talk with companies who can adapt equipment for people's specific needs.

Although sourcing equipment yourself is a cheaper option, remember that some of the equipment may not be suitable for more active people because it may break easily. Also, some equipment, such as bubble tubes, may be difficult to adapt to low voltage and can in these circumstances be a safety hazard.

Sensory aspects of the equipment

Have a clear understanding of people's sensory preferences so that you are able to buy equipment that meets the sensory needs of the people who will use the room. Take the time to analyse the equipment in terms of the sensory input it provides as well as the different ways that it can be used. Also think about how it will meet the needs of the people who will use it. The equipment checklist in Appendix 4 can be used to help work out which piece of equipment may be most suitable for the people you support. Appendix 5 contains a form that can be used to analyse the equipment in terms of senses it stimulates and ideas for use. There is also an example using the bubble tube.

Check out own environment

Equipment can often be found scattered around schools, centres or homes, so take the time to check out what is already available. In particular, review the equipment from a sensory perspective as it may have possibilities that were previously not apparent. Presents for birthdays or Christmas are another way to fund sensory equipment for an individual.

Service and maintenance

Whether a company sets up the whole room, or just provides some of the equipment, check that they have an after-sales service. Equipment invariably breaks down, so people need to know that it can be repaired as quickly as possible. If equipment is purchased from overseas, check that the local company holds spare parts or replacement equipment; otherwise, the broken equipment may be out of use for a long time while spare parts are ordered from abroad.

3
Using the Multisensory Room

This chapter is about using the multisensory room. It looks at what could be included in a procedures manual and other training topics, and it also considers general principles about usage.

Training

Once a multisensory room is set up, it is essential that training be provided if the room is to be used to its fullest extent. Remember *the equipment is only as good as the person using it.* Think about the amounts of money that can be spent on multisensory equipment. If support people are not trained in how to use the equipment and recognize its potential, a lot of effort and money may be wasted. In addition, if support people do not know how to use the equipment properly, or how to set up the room according to people's specific needs, adverse effects may occur.

One of the most common mistakes people make is to go into the multisensory room and turn on every piece of equipment. This can be very over-stimulating and people can become distressed and agitated to the extent that they can exhibit self-injurious behaviour, which is contrary to the purpose of the multisensory room.

Training should include the philosophy to be followed when using the room, how to use the individual pieces of equipment, any precautions for using the equipment, how to set up the room for different uses and how to set up the room for people's individual needs. Support people also need to know that at times it is appropriate to 'do nothing' but share the experience and observe what is happening with the person with a disability. Support people also need time to 'experience' the environment and feel positive about it. If not, their unclear/negative attitudes may be passed onto the people they support.

Procedures

Once the room has been set up, consider writing a procedures manual. The value of a procedures manual prior to using a multisensory room is that support people are clear about how the room should be used and where to go for help. The procedures manual should be part of the training package and could include information on the following.

Philosophy

- This section should define how the room should be used.

- Decide on the philosophy to be used – for example, is it a pure Snoezelen™ philosophy, or will it be used for skills training as well?

- Ensure that people are clear about why they are using the room. Too often, people are using a multisensory room with no clear idea as to why they should be there.

Eligibility

- Define who will be using the room.

- If the multisensory room is built at a specific day centre or school, decide if it will be available to people external to the organization.

Use of other facilities

- Decide if people from the wider community will be able to use other facilities such as the toilets or dining area for lunch/drinks.

- What impact will this have on the centre/school/home?

Booking the room

- Define the booking procedure.

- Nominate a person for timetabling the use of the room.

- Decide on the cost of hire.

- Decide if it is a prerequisite that people have training before using the room.

- Define the process for ongoing training.

- When people book the room, let them know if shoes have to be removed before going into the room.

Record keeping

- This should include the procedure for recording people's responses to the equipment and the environment.

- The records should reflect the aims for using the room.

- Include samples of recording forms.

Equipment – precautions and suppliers

For each piece of equipment include:

- a photograph and description

- information on how the equipment works

- guidance on the different ways the equipment can be used

- advice on precautions to be taken

- a note of where and when the equipment was purchased

- a contact number for repairs

- advice on maintenance and cleaning.

Maintaining and cleaning the environment

- Define the process for regular maintenance.

- Note the location of spare equipment – for example, globes/light bulbs, blank wheels.

- Decide if there will be a policy of one or two named people in charge of changing globes. If everyone is replacing them, there is the danger that no one will realize that the equipment is blowing globes too frequently and that there is therefore something wrong.

Reporting faults

- Describe the process to report faults. There is nothing more frustrating than going to a room and finding a piece of equipment or a switch that doesn't work.

- Nominate an appointed person to report faults, or provide a book in the room where people can record faults.

General principles

In the following list there are some general points to consider in order to ensure that a multisensory room is used effectively.

Principle	What you should do
Get to know the equipment.	Think about all the different ways the equipment can be used. Activities in the room can be linked to a person's goals and objectives as identified in planning documentation such as essential lifestyle plans/person-centred plans.
Use one piece of equipment at a time when introducing people to the multisensory room.	Initially use one piece of equipment at a time to see how much stimulation a person can process and respond to. Add more pieces of equipment if people are able to tolerate a more stimulating environment. Some people feel overwhelmed by too much sensory input. Be aware that sensory overload can result in people withdrawing or becoming very agitated.
Use continuous sensory input to help people relax.	For example, having the bubble tube going all the time can make people feel sleepy and relaxed.
Use intermittent sensory input to help people stay alert and therefore learn new skills.	Use the timer on the power box or a timer element on sensory equipment. This means that the equipment will work for a period of time and then stop. People will need to operate a switch to restart the equipment. Giving intermittent sensory input not only helps people to stay awake and alert but there is also the opportunity to teach cause and effect.
Make the multisensory room interactive, both with equipment and socially.	Offer people the opportunity to use switches to turn on equipment. Spend time with people and learn their language. Take it in turns to have a conversation using their language (e.g. mirror vocalizations, other sounds and movements).
Control the amount of stimulation presented.	Present pieces of equipment one at a time so that it is clear what people are responding to.

Remember to repeat stimuli.	Present the same piece of equipment again and over different sessions. Are responses consistent?
	Present equipment and activities in the same way each time so that people can begin to anticipate what happens next.
Give a person time to register and respond to a stimulus or piece of equipment.	Present the equipment slowly and leave it on for a few minutes to see if people notice it. If they are interested, leave it on for longer.
	Don't change the stimulus or equipment too quickly. It may take some people longer than others to notice the equipment and respond to it.
Keep a stimulus going for as long as a person is interested.	Note a person's attention span – how long will they interact with a piece of equipment before they lose interest?
Take time to make observations.	Observe a person's behaviour closely to see how they respond to equipment. Does their behaviour indicate that they are interested, disinterested or dislike the equipment?
	Observe a person's response to you. Do they notice that you are there? Are they interested in you?
Think about the time the activity takes place.	Some people take medication at lunch time that makes them drowsy, so morning sessions when people are more alert may be better for skills training or assessment. Some people get tired in the afternoon and would therefore enjoy a relaxing environment.
Activities within the multisensory room need an aim and purpose; otherwise, once the initial excitement about having new equipment wears off, people can lose interest.	Document the reasons for using the room. Keep recording forms up to date. Evaluate the recording forms and write a summary. Modify the next session based on new information.

Multisensory rooms should not be used in isolation.	Think about other sensory activities e.g. sensory cookery, sensory art, and how to use the wider community for sensory activities like visiting a sensory garden or musical concert.
The multisensory room is not a vacuum.	Think about how information gained in the multisensory room can be used in the person's life elsewhere – for example, if teaching a person cause and effect so they can turn on the bubble tube, teach them to use this skill at home by turning on their light or cassette recorder. Remember that specific skills will probably have to be taught in different locations as many people have difficulty generalizing skills learnt.
Equipment should be portable so that it can be used in different settings.	There are always other pieces of sensory equipment that can be taken into a multisensory room, or equipment can be taken from a multisensory room into another room.

Principal uses for multisensory environments

The multisensory room can be used for skills training, relaxation and leisure. Assessment is inherent in all the ways that a multisensory room is used. It is the first step in teaching skills, because it is important to know what skills people have and what environment works best for them. Assessment will also be used during relaxation to evaluate whether or not a particular environment does help a person to relax. Leisure activities are not assessed as such, but the type of leisure activity will be assessed to see if people are enjoying and participating in it.

Assessment will be considered as a separate section because there are a number of observations to be made to help determine the best way to set up a multisensory room for a particular person and which pieces of equipment they may be most motivated to interact with.

Assessment

It is recommended that support people liaise with teachers or therapists in terms of formal assessment, using their observational skills to gather appropriate data. It is often difficult to work out what interests a person with profound and multiple disabilities and therefore to engage them, either socially or with their environment. To find this out, it is important to look at self-engagement behaviours, other objects and activities people are interested in and their sensory thresholds.

SELF-ENGAGEMENT BEHAVIOURS

Many people have an inherent need to explore and experience some form of sensory stimulation. If people are unable physically to move around or are living in unstimulating environments, they may try to seek sensory stimulation from their bodies or clothes – for example, by rocking, or chewing on a jumper (i.e. self-engagement behaviours). The problem is that some people find these behaviours so absorbing that they are unaware of the stimuli in the environment around them. This makes it difficult for them to learn new skills or to interact with other people because they are so focused on the sensations they get from themselves. Interesting activities and environments need to be provided to teach people that the world around them may also be rewarding and interesting.

It is unlikely that all self-engagement behaviours can be eliminated as everyone engages in them to some degree (e.g. by jiggling a leg or chewing on a pen), and for many adults it has become a habit. However, if this behaviour is the result of seeking sensory input, it can be reduced. Providing activities and equipment that are as motivating as the sensory input people receive from their self-engagement behaviours can do this.

Analysing the types of behaviour people are exhibiting can give an indication of the type of sensory input that most interests them. For example, if a person rocks, they could be stimulated by the sense of movement. There could also be a touch component for as they rock, their clothes move with them. If people are motivated by touch and movement, they may not be interested in looking at pictures projected from the solar effects projector because this provides visual stimulation, which they are not as interested in. It would be better to offer the opportunity of moving in a leaf chair (a suspended chair in the shape of a leaf), hammock, rocking on the trampoline, or lying on an airbed, experiences which also provide touch and movement stimulation.

Vibration is a form of tactile/movement stimulation, which is very motivating for some people, so, if a person rocks or seeks other forms of tactile/movement input, they may also find a vibrating mat or massager stimulating. However, a note of caution when using vibrating equipment: do not use around the ears or chest as it can cause adverse effects.

People may also exhibit self-engagement behaviour by being preoccupied with a particular object. If they are using it in a stereotypical way – for example, twirling a shoelace or piece of thin plastic – this is self-engagement behaviour and not object engagement behaviour because the person is not exploring the sensory properties of the object or using it functionally. However, do not remove the object and give them something else to explore before first ascertaining whether or not they are using it to calm themselves. In this instance, if the object is removed, this could cause increased anxiety and other self-engagement behaviours.

One way of analysing a person's self-engagement behaviours and sensory preferences is to use the engagement background questionnaire (see Appendix 6). The self-engagement section looks at the type of behaviour a person may exhibit – for example, rocking, or swaying their head from side to side. This section also contains a 'sensory system' column, whereby the sensory system that the behaviour stimulates can be documented. For example rocking may be stimulating the senses of touch and movement and swaying the head may stimulate the sense of movement and/or vision.

When working with people with profound and multiple disabilities, it is sometimes necessary to make assumptions. For example, flicking fingers in front of the eyes could stimulate the sense of movement or the sense of vision. If people exhibit a number of behaviours, it may be possible to build up a profile so that, if all the other behaviours stimulate the sense of vision, then the finger flicking would probably be stimulating the sense of vision as well.

PREFERRED ACTIVITIES AND OBJECTS

Another way to work out what sensory system people are most interested in is to make a list of all the activities they like and dislike, and write down which sensory systems these stimulate. For example, people may like going on the swing, being on the bus, using the trampoline or swimming. All these activities have a strong movement component. It is also useful to analyse specific objects and work out the sensory properties of liked objects. For example, is the liked object smooth or rough, does it make a sound, can it be easily manipulated or is it shiny or colourful? A likes and dislikes form can be found in Appendix 7.

SENSORY THRESHOLDS

A multisensory room can be used to provide people with different sensory experiences to help replace or reduce their self-engagement behaviours. However, it is not enough to just find out what type of stimuli interests a person. It is also important to discover the intensity they like, or they will continue with their self-engagement behaviours because they find these more rewarding. This information needs to be gathered over a period of weeks or months to ensure consistency of results.

People also have different sensory thresholds so that they need differing amounts of stimulation to enable them to engage with their environment in an adaptable and functional way. Some people need lots of sensory input to be aware of their environment, but others need very little and can easily become over-stimulated. For those who get over-stimulated easily, it is important that their environment is modified so that it is structured and predictable, enabling them to make sense of what is going on. The multisensory room is one place where this is easy to do, if the room is set up and used correctly.

In terms of sensory thresholds, it is also important to work out why people are exhibiting self-engagement behaviours. Thresholds are the point at which nerves are activated by the sensations they receive. All people have different thresholds that have to be reached for the nerves to fire. For example, people have different pain thresholds, some people tolerating a lot of pain and others very little. This is the same for all the senses; therefore, a person's sensory threshold determines how much or how little sensory input they require to function effectively. Some people need lots of sensory input to be aware of their environment, but others need very little and can easily become over-stimulated.

The self-engagement behaviours, therefore, could be indicating that a person wants more sensory input, or it may be their way of indicating that they have a low tolerance to sensory input and are using the self-engagement activities as calming strategies. For example, people will often rock or hug themselves if they are anxious. They may also exhibit self-engagement behaviours in an attempt to block out extra sensory input. For example, they may make a noise, such as a constant hum or a loud yell, to drown out the other auditory stimuli that they cannot cope with. It is imperative that people have an assessment – for example, from an occupational therapist – to ensure that there is a correct understanding of self-engagement behaviours – are they indicating that a person wants more sensory input, or that they can't cope with the sensory input that already exists in their environment?

Skills development

The multisensory room is another place where people can learn to interact with objects and other people. By having a controllable environment, it can be easier to teach people skills such as cause and effect so that they can learn that they can have an effect on their environment. If someone is stimulated by the sensation of wind, they may soon learn that, if they press the switch to the fan in the multisensory room, they will feel the wind on their hands and faces. However, if they press the button on the hand drier in the local toilets, there may be other people using the hand driers at the same time, so it is difficult for them to work out what they have done. Having said that, once people understand cause and effect, it is important for them to use that skill in all activities of daily living. To extend the effectiveness from the experiences of the multisensory room, teach people to use the hand driers in public toilets, or turn on a fan in their bedrooms on hot days.

In a multisensory room, people require time to explore the environment and equipment. Once a person has indicated they like something, they can be taught how to access it. This is either through promoting communication, so that they can indicate to support people that they want a certain object if they cannot reach it, or through teaching people how to use a switch to activate an object. Through this process, people develop skills and gain control over their environment.

The following sections look at some of the skills that can be taught in a multisensory room. However, the room is only one vehicle that can be used to teach skills.

DEVELOPMENT OF VISUAL SKILLS

People with profound and multiple disabilities can have visual impairments, but it is sometimes difficult to work out what exactly they can see. A multisensory room can be darkened and light sources controlled to see whether people respond to light. People who do not seem to respond to light in the natural environment will sometimes become still or look towards a light source in the multisensory room because of the contrast between the darkened room and a light source such as a torch or spotlight.

Lights can be shone at different distances close up or far away and also in different places – for example, above a person or to the side to encourage them to look around their environment.

Some people may not appear to be using their vision. If people do not seem to respond to the light, experiment with moving it in their peripheral vision (i.e. to the side) as people can sometimes notice a moving object better than a stationary one.

If using lights to develop tracking skills (i.e. watching a light moving around a room), remember to move the light slowly. If the light is moved too quickly, people may not have time to find it and follow it before it moves again.

DEVELOPMENT OF OBJECT ENGAGEMENT SKILLS

Object engagement skills involve teaching people how to interact with objects rather than just their bodies (self-engagement behaviours). The first step in developing interaction with objects is to help people notice the objects and then present the objects in a way that motivates the people to want to interact with them.

By interacting with objects, people can become more interested in exploring their external environment. To find objects that motivate people to explore, use objects that appeal to their sensory preferences. Determine this by analysing the sensory input they are seeking from their bodies or clothes.

Once a person has found an object they want to explore, this object can be used to teach cause and effect to assist people in developing control over aspects of their environment. Having control over the environment can increase motivation to explore it.

Brinker and Lewis (1982) state: 'handicapped infants may begin to lose interest in a world which they do not expect to control' (p.164). The longer they are unable to control their environment, the less motivated they are to try in the future. This may also lead to an increase in self-engagement behaviour (e.g. rocking), which they can control. This is as applicable to adults as it is to children.

In developing the concept of cause and effect, people will be required to understand that their actions have an effect on their environment – for example, activating a switch turns on the bubble tube. If a person does not understand this, position the switch close to them so that they can accidentally activate the switch through the course of their normal movements. In time, they may notice that something interesting happens, even if they do not understand that they have caused it to happen. Co-active assistance can be used if people do not reach out to use the switch. Co-active assistance involves guiding a person's movements to activate a switch. Remember when working co-actively to support and guide the movement from the elbow, while supporting the hand at the wrist to operate it. As people learn to use the switch, move it further away from them so they actively have to reach to operate it.

Offering people choices about which piece of equipment to use can further develop interaction with objects. When offering choices, start with a choice between two pieces of equipment. Use items that are very different from each other in terms of sensory input – for example, the bubble tube or vibrating bed.

To develop further cognitive skills, colour code the switches to see if people can learn which colour operates which piece of equipment. This can also be used to teach colour recognition. Make sure there is consistency with using the same coloured switches for the same pieces of equipment.

DEVELOPMENT OF COMMUNICATION SKILLS

To develop communication skills, opportunities need to be available for people to interact with their peers as well as support people. Time is required for support people to understand the unique ways people communicate, and activities need to be presented in a way that people understand.

Opportunities to interact with peers

The multisensory room is another environment where people have the opportunity to practise interacting not just with objects but with other people as well. As Hulsegge and Verheul (1987) state: 'Most important are the interpersonal contacts. These can never be substituted by machines or effects. And this will always have to be the starting-point from which we can share the sensations of Snoezelen™' (p.14).

As with any environment, create opportunities for people to interact and strengthen relationships with one another. Setting up a 'greetings' routine, whereby people are given the time and opportunity to say 'hello' to each other, can assist in developing relationships. People use lots of different ways to say hello. Some people use sounds, some a look and smile, others use touch or wave their hands.

To facilitate interactions, people need to be near each other and helped to be made aware that the other person is there. Some people may not notice others if they are sitting on the other side of the room. If people are unable to move independently, help them move close to someone and encourage looking at or reaching out to the person next to them.

Time to interact with support people

Often people are rushed and focused on getting a particular task done. The multisensory room can be used as a space where there is no particular agenda but the time is used to just enjoy being with each other. This time can be used to communicate with someone in their own language, which may be sounds or movements. Wait for the person to communicate in their own way and then respond using their sounds or movements. Wait again, and see if they respond to you. This time of showing mutual interest in each other is an important foundation for interaction. For more information on this technique, refer to Nind and Hewitt's (2001) book on intensive interaction.

Also think about different ways in which people can identify support staff. Not everyone will understand a person's spoken name, so have a personal object reference – for example, a special key ring, bangle, watch and/or a particular aftershave/shampoo – that represents you.

Time to observe how people communicate

Take time to observe how people indicate whether or not they like a particular piece of equipment. Use the information to compile a personal communication dictionary (PCD). A PCD is a way of recording a person's individual responses to equipment and then noting what they think it means. Everyone working with the person must agree on the meaning of the responses so that everyone interacts with that person in a consistent manner. An example of a PCD form can be found in Appendix 8.

Level of communication

Think about a person's level of communication and set up the environment so that they understand what is going on. For example, if they are offered the choice of which piece of equipment they want to use, what is the best way to illustrate the choice? Do people need object symbols to represent the equipment and the multisensory room? An object symbol is a three-dimensional representation of the real object or activity (see Figure 3.1). If an object symbol of the

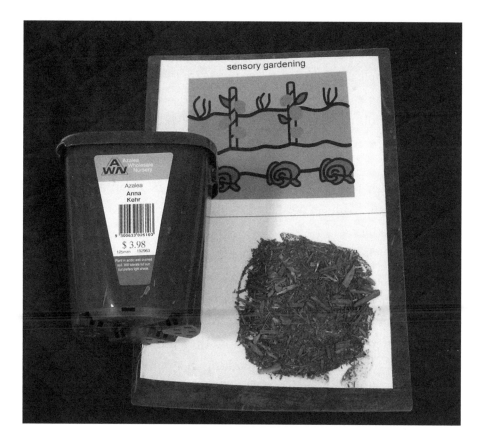

Figure 3.1 Object symbol for gardening

multisensory room is used, offer it to people to explore before going to the room, so that they can begin to anticipate that they are going there.

Some people may recognize photographs, so take photographs of the pieces of equipment so that they can use these to make choices. Other people can use pictographs or line drawings to represent the equipment.

It is often useful to have a wall or panel of Velcro®-compatible material so that photographs or line drawings can be displayed. A pictorial or object symbol timetable can also be used, so that people know when they are going to the multisensory room. A finish box, which is a box used to indicate that an activity has ended, can be added to the timetable. Thus, when the session has ended, the object symbol or photograph of the sensory room is placed in the finish box.

Relaxation

People can indicate through their mood and behaviour whether or not they are calm or agitated. Some people may become anxious or annoyed if there is too much noise or there are too many people close to them. If the multisensory room is set up to be multifunctional, it can be used as a space where people can relax and experience reduced stimulation. Some people get more agitated at certain times of the day, and the multisensory room can be used to help them relax so that they may then be able to join in other structured group activities.

When setting up the room for relaxation, the aim is not to set up an environment where people go to sleep and are then left. Set up a peaceful time where people can unwind. This means that support people need to be there to observe people, to see if and when they do relax. Observe to see how long it takes for people to relax. If people are not relaxing, the equipment in the room may need to be adjusted so that they can.

Some people feel uncomfortable in their wheelchairs for a long period of time. The multisensory room gives them an interesting environment to interact with while experiencing different positions such as lying on mats or over wedges.

At other times, people may already be calm, but the aim may be to create a peaceful time that you can both share. There is the opportunity for people to develop trust and understanding because of the quality one-to-one time spent with each other in the room. Watch to see which piece of equipment a person is attending to, and record how they indicate that they are happy and relaxed.

Remember, when working in a multisensory room it is important *not to put on all the equipment at once*. This is especially true when trying to help a person relax. A multitude of stimuli presented at the same time can be over-stimulating. It is easy to create an atmosphere for relaxation by dimming the lights and using soothing music, relaxing essential oils and maybe one light effect as a focal point. However, remember to check that people can tolerate these different stimuli.

When conducting massage in the multisensory room, remember that it is an interactive process. It is more than just rubbing oils and lotions on people's hands and feet. Look to see if people are enjoying the experience, which part of the body they prefer to have massaged, which oil/lotion they prefer, how long they can tolerate a massage and the level of intensity they prefer. An interactive massage sequence can be found in Sanderson and Harrison's (1996) book on aromatherapy and massage for people with learning difficulties.

Leisure

One way of using the multisensory room for leisure is to set up theme environments for people to explore. Themes are a useful way to help structure the environment. They can either be set up in a corner of a room, or the multisensory room can be set up as a theme room, incorporating the equipment that is already in there.

When planning theme environments, think about religious, seasonal and holiday events and plan themes around them – for example, Easter, Christmas, winter, spring, summer and autumn. Also think about different cultural stories such as aboriginal tales and major events in people's lives such as birthdays. Themes can run throughout a person's day or week. For example, places can be visited to gather items for the theme, art and craft activities can be used to make items for the theme room, and cookery activities can be used to incorporate the taste part of a theme, as this may not be appropriate to do in the actual multisensory room.

It is useful to think about theme environments in terms of the different senses and how these senses can be incorporated into a theme. This idea is expanded on in Chapter 6 where the information on different themes and stories have been divided up under the senses of touch, movement, seeing, hearing, smell and taste.

A multisensory room can also be set up as a multisensory theatre where interactive sensory-focused stories take place. In the course of telling different stories, the space can be used creatively and flexibly as a vehicle to change the set-up of the room and keep it interesting to explore. Start with some basic props, use them in different ways and add to them to create a limitless number of themes and stories. Ultimately, these stories could take place in mainstream theatres, but the multisensory room is a space to try out new ideas.

By using the space for a sensory story or theme, multisensory experiences can be provided and the trap of providing people with too much stimulation at once avoided. This is because only the piece of equipment that is relevant to the story at that time is used, rather than turning everything on at once. It also provides the time and opportunity for people to interact with the equipment, turning on and experiencing pieces of equipment as the story unfolds. These stories can appeal to all ability levels, because some people may be able to follow the story while others experience its sensory components. Refer to Chapter 6 for examples of sensory stories. There is also an example of a story outline showing how to incorporate different pieces of multisensory equipment into the story (Appendix 9).

To enable people to learn the sequence of events during the story and to begin to anticipate what happens next, tell the story the same way for a number of weeks. The story can also be used to provide a structure for a variety of activities – for example, people can bake and taste items related to the story, or make the props for the story.

Another way to make use of the multisensory room for leisure purposes is to use it to recount a trip people have had, or funny events that have occurred in their lives. Collect items from the outing that can be explored at a later date. Also take digital photographs of trips and project them onto the wall via a computer, or create a wheel for the solar projector so that the images can be projected onto the wall. To make projector wheels, refer to Appendix 10 or go to Richard Hirstwood's website on www.multi-sensory-room.co.uk. This website also has many ideas on how to use other equipment in a multisensory room.

Example of how to use the multisensory room in a structured way

The previous section discussed the different uses for the multisensory room. This next section sets out in detail how to run a specific session in the multisensory room, where the aim is to find out what sensory experiences or equipment people like.

1. Prior to going into the multisensory room, offer people an object symbol that represents the room, to touch and look at, so that they know where they are going.

2. Have a greeting sequence using a personal cue (such as a bracelet or ring) or touch cue (a particular way a person is touched) to help people recognize who they are working with.

3. Stand back and observe what people are doing in the multisensory room – for example,

    o Are they showing self-engagement behaviours such as rocking or finger sucking?

    o Do these behaviours stop when the equipment is on?

    o Do they show an interest in the equipment?

4. Turn off the equipment and observe whether or not people notice the equipment is off. Do their self-engagement behaviours start again?

5. Turn the equipment back on – do they re-orientate and notice it is back on?

6. If a person shows an interest in a particular piece of equipment, use it to promote communication or teach them to use a switch to turn it on themselves.

7. Move onto another piece of equipment.

8. At the end of the session, record findings from your observations, noting which pieces of equipment people liked, how you know this and what sensory system(s) the equipment stimulated.

PART TWO

MULTISENSORY EQUIPMENT

4

Introduction to Part Two

This part examines the multisensory equipment. Chapter 5 looks at some common pieces of commercially available equipment and suggests different ways in which they can be used. By doing this, it is possible to discover valuable information about people's interests. For example, it may be that a person is interested in the bubble tube, not because of the visual aspect but because they can feel the vibrations from the pump or hear the water gurgling up the tube. On subsequent occasions, different pieces of equipment could be used to see if there is a pattern – for example, does the person always show a 'like' response when the equipment is used to stimulate the touch sense? Remember to use the same piece of equipment more than once to ensure that people really do like it.

Chapter 5 will not go into detailed descriptions of the multisensory equipment, but will analyse common items in terms of the senses they stimulate. Equipment is grouped under a main sense, but a lot of the equipment can be used in multisensory ways. The sense of taste has been omitted, because it is more appropriate to offer this stimulus at other times such as during sensory cookery or meal times. Liaise with a speech pathologist to ensure that people are safe to eat the foods and drinks suggested, and remember to check for any allergies or special dietary requirements.

Some of the activities suggest using essential oils. Consult with an aromatherapist about the most appropriate oils to use, and be aware of any con-traindications.

Where applicable, cheaper pieces of equipment have been described or mentioned as a less costly alternative, as well as ideas for incorporating sensory activities within everyday life. This means that anyone can set up a multisensory environment be it in a home, school or service, and it is not necessary to set up a specific room.

Each piece of equipment has the following information:

- a brief description
- precautions – be sure to check all recommendations by the manufacturers and ensure that the room or equipment have circuit breakers or safety switches
- aims for using the equipment

- how to use the equipment to stimulate the different senses

- where appropriate, a list of other ways to use the equipment

- cheaper and everyday alternatives where applicable.

For more detailed descriptions of equipment and further ideas, refer to *A Practical Guide to the Use of Multisensory Rooms* by Richard Hirstwood and Mark Grey (1995).

Chapter 6 offers some ideas for theme and story development in relation to the pieces of equipment. Each story or theme has the following information:

- the equipment required

- how to use the story/theme to stimulate the different senses.

In addition, two scripts are included to show how a particular story can be represented.

5

Using the Multisensory Equipment

This chapter, which offers ideas for multisensory equipment, is divided into four sections, as follows:

1. Touch

2. Movement

3. Seeing

4. Hearing

5. Smell

Activities
TOUCH

VIBRATING AND VIBROACOUSTIC BEDS

Description

These are made of soft play mats mounted onto a platform. The platforms can be made to different heights and with space under them so that they can be used with a portable hoist. They can be built to be switch-operated, with a timer and an intensity control so that people can experience very mild to intense vibrations. Where possible, purchase a bed that vibrates in sections, because people may tolerate vibrations on their legs but not like the sensations up around their shoulders. Some of these beds only vibrate, but others have speakers within them so that they can be linked up to a sound system or microphone to respond to the beat from music or vocalizations (i.e. vibroacoustic beds). A variation on the vibroacoutic bed is the vibroacoustic beanbag which also responds to the beat from music (see Figure 2.6 on p.34).

PRECAUTIONS

- Never leave people on a vibrating mat for long periods of time. They can become over-stimulated by the vibrations and agitated or incontinent as a result.

- Where possible, purchase a bed or mat that has an intensity control. Some people may not be able to tolerate intense vibrations, but may enjoy a mild sensation.

- Do not use any vibrating equipment around the ears or chest as it may adversely affect some people.

- Do not use massage mats or seats for more than 30 minutes, because extensive use could cause the product to overheat.

- Ensure that the hand-control unit is in the OFF position before plugging the massage mat into the wall socket.

- Individuals with pacemakers should consult a doctor before using the massage equipment.

- Do not use under a blanket as overheating can occur.

- Always read the warnings and safety instructions that come with any equipment.

- When cleaning the mats, only use a soft, slightly damp sponge. Do not allow water to come into contact with the hand unit.

Copyright © Scope (Vic.) Ltd 2008

Aims for using the equipment

- To provide tactile/movement stimulation in the form of vibration.
- To provide auditory stimulation.
- To provide a relaxing environment.
- To arouse a person (depending on the intensity of the vibrations, a person will become aroused or relaxed).
- To teach cause and effect.
- To promote communication skills (i.e people indicate when they want the mat/bed turned back on).
- To provide an opportunity to express likes and dislikes.
- To provide an opportunity to make choices.
- To provide an object of interest (many people appear to be motivated by vibration).

How to use the equipment to stimulate the different senses

Touch

- Place a person on the mat/beanbag/seat.
- Experiment with the different intensities to see which ones people prefer (e.g. Do they prefer a very subtle vibration or a strong vibration?).

Movement

- As the person is vibrated on the mat/seat, they will also experience a sense of movement.

Seeing

- Not applicable.
- However, the mat/bed can be used in conjunction with other equipment (e.g. place a person on a vibrating mat and project an image onto the wall for them to look at, or drape the fibre-optic spray around them).

Hearing

- Using the vibroacoustic beds and beanbags, experiment with different types of music. Which types do people prefer? Do they like soft music that gives subtle vibrations or heavy rock that gives intense ones?
- If a mat has a sound headpiece, do people like the sounds from the headpiece? Which do they prefer?

Smell

- Not applicable.
- However, the equipment can be used with other equipment (e.g. as people are relaxing on the vibrating mat, have the aroma of relaxing oils blown into the room).

 Copyright © Scope (Vic.) Ltd 2008

Other ways to use the equipment

- Try different positions – do people prefer to lie on a mat or sit up and feel the vibrations through a seat or back cushion?

- Use the massage mat on people's feet and hands.

- Use the heat element from a massage mat – do people prefer this to the vibrations?

Cheaper and everyday alternatives

- An interactive cushion can be linked up to sound systems and computers so that it responds to the beat from music/sound from computer games or CD/DVD players. The newer versions also come with a vibration-only option.

- Use a vibrating belt massager under the corner of an air mattress to create a 'vibrating bed'.

- Buy massage mats from department and electrical stores. Some are three-quarter length body mats, which can be rolled up for storage. Others are seat or back cushions. They all come with a controller to control the intensity of the vibration. Some have a heat element as part of the mat and others have a sound system built into the headpiece, which plays relaxing sounds such as the noise of a waterfall or bird calls. People find them very motivating and they are portable so they can easily be used in different locations.

- Buy a vibrating snake/massage tube. These are coloured tubes with black caps at each end and they are also known as massage belts. They are battery-operated and can be switch-adapted so that people use a switch to control the vibrations of the snake. Vibrations are felt more intensely if held in the middle rather than at the ends. The vibrating snake can be placed on a table or bench to increase the sounds of the vibration. Some people are more interested in listening to the noise of it vibrating on the bench, or watching it move as it vibrates. Make the snake more colourful by covering it with shiny fabric.

- Instead of buying an expensive vibrating bed, use the money to put together a vibrating sensory box. Collect together as many different items as possible to provide a variety of experiences (e.g. vibrating key rings, animals, massagers, balls).

- Hold onto a blender, feel a food processor or put your hands on a table to feel the vibrations from the electrical equipment while making a drink, dip or cake.

- Buy an electric toothbrush.

- Buy an electric shaver.

- Buy a variety of hand-held neck and head massagers.

Copyright © Scope (Vic.) Ltd 2008

FANS

Description

A table fan is a cheap and versatile piece of equipment. Some people respond to the feel of the wind from the fan on their face or body. Others are motivated by the sound of wind chimes or streamers, which are moved by the wind from the fan.

PRECAUTIONS

- Ensure that the fan has a fine grid around the blades so that people cannot put their fingers in them.

- In some situations, the fan will need to be secured to a shelf or wall.

Aims for using the equipment

- To provide tactile stimulation (breeze from the fan).
- To give auditory stimulation when directed onto the wind chimes or foil streamers.
- To provide visual stimulation – watching items move in the breeze.
- To motivate a person to attend.
- To practise switching skills and cause and effect (the equipment can be switch-adapted or plugged into a power box).
- To teach cause and effect, using communication; people will either look at you or vocalize when they want the fan back on.
- To foster working in partnership with one's peers – taking it in turns to use the fan.
- To provide an opportunity to express likes and dislikes.
- To offer an opportunity to make choices.
- To create a relaxing environment by directing the fan onto small, quiet wind chimes or streamers that gently flow.
- To increase awareness of body parts by directing the wind to different parts of the body.

How to use the equipment to stimulate the different senses

Touch

- Feel the breeze on the face/limbs. Remember to vary the intensity of the breeze. Some people will like a light breeze, others will prefer a stronger one.
- Attach streamers/ribbons to the fan and feel them being blown from the fan onto the face/limbs (some people may find this light touch irritating).

Movement

- Encourage people to reach out and use the switch or feel the streamers and other items moving in the breeze.

 Copyright © Scope (Vic.) Ltd 2008

Seeing

- Watch streamers that are attached to the fan – close up.
- Watch streamers/foil in the distance as the breeze from the fan blows on them.

Hearing

- Listen to wind chimes as the breeze blows on them. Think about the different sounds created by using different wind chimes (e.g. bamboo wind chimes, small bells).
- Make your own wind chimes from old spoons.
- Think about the sounds that different materials make as the wind blows on them (e.g. cloth streamers, foil streamers, cellophane streamers).

Smell

- Attach scented ribbons to the fan so that the aroma is blown around when the fan is turned on.

Other ways to use the equipment

- Set up an individual sensory environment using a beach tent. Attach bells or streamers to the tent. A person can sit or lie in the tent and use a switch to turn on the fan. This will then set the bells and steamers moving.
- Suspend wind chimes from ceiling grids, hooks on the wall, activity arches or individual arches attached to a wheelchair tray. Use the breeze from a fan to set them moving.
- Direct a spotlight onto the chimes to highlight the movement and shadows created when the wind from the fan blows on them (Helen Dilkes).
- Glue fluorescent streamers onto a hoop and suspend from the ceiling. Put on the UV light and attach the fan to a power box. Sit under the hoop and turn the fan on. People can experience the steamers swirling around them. Beware of precautions when using UV light.
- Direct the fan towards a lace curtain/white streamers so that people can watch the lace/streamers moving.
- Attach shower hooks onto the lace curtain and suspend it from a metal/wooden pole. The curtain can then be bunched together or pulled across a room or corner of a room. Use the lace curtain or a curtain of white streamers as a projection screen, project slides/solar projector onto it and direct the fan onto that. The lace/streamers will then appear to be moving colours.
- Direct the fan onto different parts of the body.Fans CONTINUED

Cheaper and everyday alternatives

- Go outside on a blustery day. Wrap up in warm clothing and feel the wind on your face, in your hair. Feel your scarf moving in the breeze.
- Feel the warm air from a hand drier.
- Feel warm/cold air from a hair drier.
- Visit a hairdresser's for a wash and blow dry.
- Use a small battery-operated fan (used to dry nail polish).

Copyright © Scope (Vic.) Ltd 2008

TACTILE WALLS

Description

These can be bought commercially or made yourself. They are usually one piece of board or individual panels with different textures. Some panels also vibrate or have fans, echo tubes or lights as well as textures. The textures may be mop heads, lamb's wool, paint rollers, broom heads, different pieces of material, panels with bird seed, koosh balls and strings of beads – the list is endless and is only limited by your imagination. Some of these panels are also linked to a keyboard. The following photograph (see Figure 5.1) shows a tactile wall.

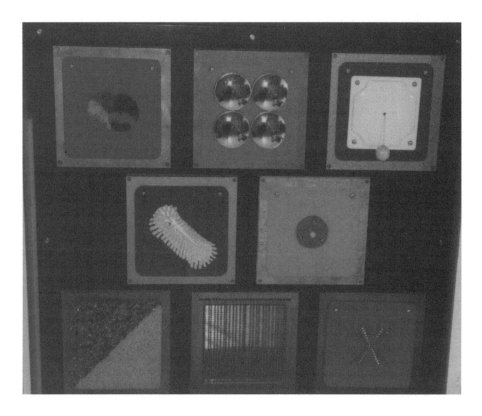

Figure 5.1 Tactile wall

If you are having tactile wall panels made (see Figure 5.2), ensure that they are a standard size so that they can either be used on the wall or in an activity table.

When purchasing a tactile wall or making it yourself, ensure that there are not too many different things on the wall, because this can be quite confusing for some people. It is better to have a few large areas of the same texture than lots of little ones with different textures.

PRECAUTIONS

- Ensure that all the pieces are firmly attached.
- Think about how to keep the items clean.

Copyright © Scope (Vic.) Ltd 2008

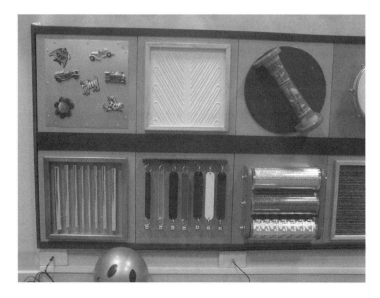

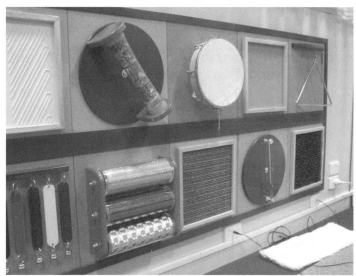

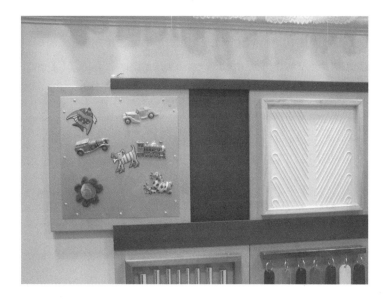

Figure 5.2 Tactile panels

Aims for using the equipment

- To provide tactile stimulation (different textures and vibration if vibration panels are included on the wall).
- To provide auditory stimulation (sound of different textures [e.g. sand paper, metal beads]).
- To provide visual stimulation as some of the textures may reflect light (e.g. holographic panels). Some tactile walls can also be purchased that have coloured acrylic panels. These walls could be mounted in windows to allow light through the coloured panels to produce bright smudges of light on the floor. Just make sure that having these colours and textures isn't over-stimulating for people.
- To motivate a person to explore.
- To provide an object of interest that a person can share with another person.
- To provide an opportunity to express likes and dislikes in terms of different textures.
- To provide an opportunity to make choices about which panels to explore.
- To practise switching skills and teach cause and effect if linked to a keyboard.

How to use the equipment to stimulate the different senses

Touch

- Feel the different textures.

Movement

- Encourage people to reach out and feel the different textures.

Seeing

- Look at the different textures and colour contrast.

Hearing

- Listen to the sounds made by touching the different textures.
- Listen to the sounds made when using an echo tube that is part of a tactile wall.

Smell

- Incorporate a panel with an air freshener, a pocket which holds cotton wool and essential oil, or attach potpourri to one of the wall panels.

Other ways to use the equipment

- Some commercially bought tactile walls are linked up to a keyboard so that, when a textured panel is pressed, it will create a note or chord. The unit is also switch accessible so that the switch operates the keyboard rather than the panels.
- Position the tactile wall near the floor so that people can lie down and feel the tactile panels with their hands or feet.
- Design tactile wall panels that can be taken off and used as tabletop inserts.

 Copyright © Scope (Vic.) Ltd 2008

Cheaper and everyday alternatives

- Make a tactile wall yourself.
- Make up a tactile book. Use thick card for the pages and glue or velcro different textures onto the pages.
- Write a book about a person or think about an event a person has been to (e.g. a train ride to visit a farm, a bus trip to a park). Add textures to the storybook such as sheep's wool, twigs and leaves.
- Make up a tactile cushion using different materials. Sew loops onto the cushion to add different textured objects. Make tactile cushions that include pockets for potpourri and other scents.
- Use a strip of Velcro®-compatible material and stick different textures onto the strip.
- Make up tactile armchair covers so that people can explore the different textures on the arms of chairs.
- Think about different textures that can be used in the bathroom and bedroom (e.g. loophas, face scrubs with gritty textures, scourers, pumice stones, massage gloves).
- Buy a massage shower head.
- Visit a masseur.
- Buy a hessian floor mat (see Figure 5.3). Feel the hessian or use it as a base to attach other items.
- Dry yourself with towels that have been warmed up in the tumble drier.
- Wrap yourself in different textured materials. Have a massage with different textures.

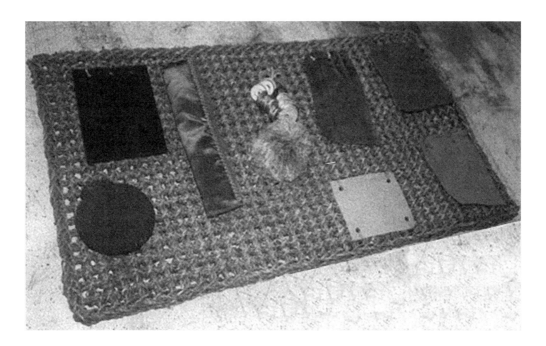

Figure 5.3 Hessian mat

Copyright © Scope (Vic.) Ltd 2008

BALL POOLS

Description

These are areas created with soft play walls and filled with hollow plastic balls. Usually the balls are coloured; however, the area can be filled with white balls. The white balls are effective when light is projected onto them. People can sink in among the balls and enjoy a total tactile experience.

Variations to the ball pool are the ball dumper and ball sorter. The ball dumper (see Figure 5.4) collects balls in a container above the ball pool. A switch is then operated to dump the balls into the ball pool.

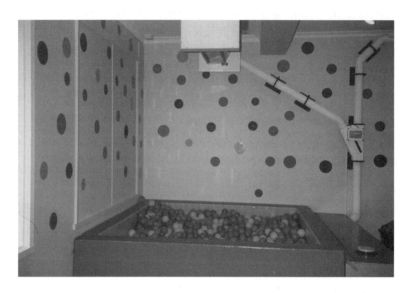

Figure 5.4 Ball dumper

The ball sorter (see Figure 5.5) is used to sort the balls into different colours – this is also switch operated.

It is imperative that the ball pool is emptied and cleaned on a regular basis. The easiest way to do this is to put the balls in nets and wash them in the nets. Wipe down the soft play pool with disinfectant.

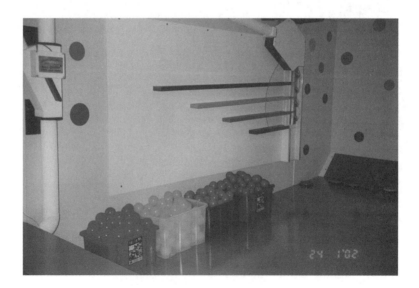

Figure 5.5 Ball sorter

 Copyright © Scope (Vic.) Ltd 2008

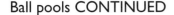

PRECAUTIONS

- Think about how people will get into and out of the ball pool – you do not want to damage your back lifting people. Use a ceiling or portable hoist.

- If a ceiling hoist is not available, have a platform made that fits the ball pool so that a portable hoist can be used. Ensure that the ball pool is securely attached to the platform.

- Some people may not be able to hold themselves up in the ball pool. They can sink under the balls, which can be a very frightening experience.

- Balls being dumped from an overhead ball dumper may scare a person.

- Some people may find the ball sorter and ball cascade very noisy and become upset and distressed.

- Remember to clean the balls and pool regularly.

- If draping a fibre-optic spray over the balls, remember to keep the light source out of the ball pool.

Aims for using the equipment

- To provide tactile stimulation.
- To provide auditory stimulation using the ball dumper.
- To provide visual stimulation, watching the balls.
- To alert or calm a person.
- To teach cause and effect – using the switch to sort or dump the balls.
- To encourage communication – do people want the balls dumped again?
- To encourage people to hold the different types of balls.
- To provide an opportunity to express likes and dislikes.
- To provide an opportunity to make choices.

How to use the equipment to stimulate the different senses

Touch

- Offer people different balls to feel.
- Immerse people in the balls.

Copyright © Scope (Vic.) Ltd 2008

Movement

- Encourage people to move themselves or parts of their body (e.g. arm, leg, hand, foot) in the ball pool.

Seeing

- Look at the different coloured balls.
- Watch the balls raining down from the ball dumper. People do not have to be in the ball pool but can operate the switch to release the balls from outside the ball pool.

Hearing

- Observe people as they listen to the rustle made by the balls in the pool.
- Observe people as they listen to the noise created by the ball sorter and ball dumper.

Smell

- Not applicable.

Other ways to use the equipment

- Add different textured and sized balls to the ball pool.
- If using white coloured balls, use the surface as a projection screen. Project different coloured images onto the balls or different coloured spotlights. Link the spotlights to a switch so that people can turn the lights on or off.
- Fill the ball pool with white materials and project different coloured lights onto them.
- Suspend netting over the ball pool and direct a fan onto it, or project images onto the netting.
- Ask people to select certain colours or numbers of balls.
- Ask people to pass the balls to one another.
- Hide different objects in the ball pool for people to find.
- Use the ball sorter to practise colour recognition.
- Use the ball dumper as a game – someone to sit in the ball pool and someone else to sit outside and operate the switch to dump the balls on people in the ball pool.

Cheaper and everyday alternatives

- Make your own ball pool using a paddling pool or children's oyster/turtle shell and fill it with different types of balls or different textures (e.g. shredded paper, different types of material).
- Create a corner unit that you can fill with shredded paper and different types of materials.
- Go for a swim or visit the hydro pool.
- Have a spa or jacuzzi.

Copyright © Scope (Vic.) Ltd 2008

FOOTSPAS

Description

Footspas are containers with a textured base and motor that vibrates the unit. They are filled with water, which vibrates when the motor is turned on. They can be purchased from many retail outlets, which is cheaper than buying them from companies selling multisensory equipment. They are a cheap and often very motivating piece of equipment.

PRECAUTION

- General care should be taken because they are powered by electricity and used with water.

Aims for using the equipment

- To provide tactile stimulation (different temperatures, water and vibrations).
- To provide auditory stimulation (hum from the vibrations).
- To provide visual stimulation (bubbles).
- To provide olfactory stimulation (scented bubbles).
- To provide a relaxing activity.
- To teach cause and effect and promote communication skills (i.e. people indicate to you when they want the vibrations turned back on).
- To provide an opportunity to express likes and dislikes.
- To provide an opportunity to make choices.
- To provide an object of interest (many people appear to be motivated by vibration).

How to use the equipment to stimulate the different senses

Touch

- Fill the footspa with warm water and turn on the vibrations. Experiment with the different intensities of vibration and water temperatures.

Movement

- Move hands/feet gently in the water and on towels when drying hands/feet.

Seeing

- Add bubbles to the footspa using bubble bath.

Hearing

- Observe people as they listen to the hum of the footspa.

Copyright © Scope (Vic.) Ltd 2008

Smell

- Observe people when different scents or aromas are added to the water.

Other ways to use the equipment

- Use the footspa with an object to promote communication (e.g. ask people to give you the bubble bath, or to look at the bottle if they want it added to the footspa).
- Use the footspa with hands.
- Use the footspa as part of a foot programme. After the footspa, dry feet with a warm fluffy towel and apply different foot lotions.
- Make you own foot lotions to use after the footspa.
- Use different textures to dry feet.
- Fill the footspa with different textures rather than water.
- If a person is unable to use the dial on the footspa link it up to a power box and use a switch to turn on the footspa.

Cheaper and everyday alternatives

- Go for a pedicure.
- Have a foot massage.
- Soak your feet in warm water with bubble bath or essential oils.
- Have a paddle at the beach.

Copyright © Scope (Vic.) Ltd 2008

Activities
MOVEMENT

LEAF CHAIRS

Description

The leaf chair is a white padded seat shaped like a leaf, which gives support and provides movement stimulation (see Figure 2.18 p.46). It can be suspended from the ceiling or a freestanding frame. If using a freestanding frame, be aware that it does take up a lot of room. If suspended from the ceiling, ensure that the ceiling is strong enough to support it.

PRECAUTIONS

- Ensure that the leaf chair is safely secured to the freestanding frame or ceiling.

- When transferring people into the chair, remember that, because it swings, it is not necessarily stable and may move away when you try and sit in it. Find some way of securing the leaf chair – for example, by strapping it to the frame while transferring.

- Ensure that people are secure in the chair and won't fall out. Some people may require a safety belt.

- Do not leave people unsupervised.

- Do not use strong solvent or abrasive cleaners as they can damage the vinyl. Use a soft, non-abrasive cloth and soap or a gentle detergent to clean.

Aims for using the equipment

- To provide movement stimulation.
- To provide tactile stimulation (e.g. feel the padded chair).
- To use as a prop in a sensory theme.
- For relaxation.

How to use the equipment to stimulate the different senses

Touch

- Lie in the chair. Put different textured mats on the seat.

Movement

- Gently move in the chair.

Copyright © Scope (Vic.) Ltd 2008

Seeing

- Not applicable – unless suspending items above the chair.

Hearing

- Not applicable – unless moving the chair gently to music.

Smell

- Not applicable

Other ways to use the equipment

- Place different textures on the seat (e.g. lamb's wool).
- Suspend netting over the frame of the leaf chair. Project different images onto the netting or hang items over it.
- Drape the fibre-optic spray over the leaf chair.
- Project the solar projector onto the chair (take care not to shine it into people's eyes).
- Use the leaf chair in a relaxing setting.

Cheaper and everyday alternatives

- Buy a garden swing seat – however, be aware that they provide minimal postural support. Also check that it is sturdy enough to withstand use from many people.
- Buy a hammock.
- Swing at the park. There arc a number of wheelchair swings now available in public parks.
- Go for a bus, train or car ride.
- Ride a horse or ride in a cart pulled by a horse.
- Listen to music and dance.
- Join a wheelchair dancing group.
- Use a rocking chair.

Copyright © Scope (Vic.) Ltd 2008

HAMMOCKS

Description

These are made from canvas or rope and are available in lying or seated positions. They can be bought from a variety of commercial outlets – for example, garden centres, community aid abroad shops. When buying a hammock, make sure that it has enough depth so that people can sink into it and are not in danger of falling out. Some hammocks come with a freestanding frame.

PRECAUTIONS

- Ensure that the hammock has a close mesh; otherwise, people can get their fingers caught in the netting.

- Ensure that the hammock is stable before transferring someone into it.

- Ensure that people are secure in the hammock.

- Ensure that the ceiling can take the weight of the hammock and the person in it.

- Make sure that the hammock is installed correctly and follow manufacturers' guidelines.

Aims for using the equipment

- To provide movement stimulation.
- To provide tactile stimulation – the feel of the mesh/cloth of the hammock.
- To use as a prop in a sensory theme.
- For relaxation.

How to use the equipment to stimulate the different senses

Touch

- Lie/sit in the hammock. Use different textures to line the hammock.

Movement

- Gently move in the hammock.

Seeing

- Not applicable – unless suspending items to look at.

Copyright © Scope (Vic.) Ltd 2008

Hearing

- Not applicable – unless moving the hammock in time to music.

Smell

- Not applicable – unless lavender bags are placed in the hammock.

Other ways to use the equipment

- Use the frame to suspend netting over the hammock. Project different images onto the netting or hang things over it.
- Drape the fibre-optic spray around the hammock.
- Use the hammock in a relaxing setting.
- Use the hammock to help a person become more tolerant to touch. Consult with an occupational therapist on how to set up this sort of programme.

Copyright © Scope (Vic.) Ltd 2008

WATER BEDS/WATER CHAIRS

Description

Water beds are covered with vinyl soft play material and can come with supporting walls that help maintain their shape. They can also be heated. Some of the water beds incorporate a sound system so that people can feel the beat of the music through the water mattress. Others have microphones attached so that people can experience the vibrations from their voices through the water in the beds.

Water chairs come as relaxing lounge chairs. They are available as reclining chairs.

PRECAUTIONS

- Because these items are mats or cushions surrounding water, they can become punctured and the water leak out.

- Ensure that sharp objects are kept away from the water bed or chair to prevent punctures.

- If using a lilo, remember to keep enough air in it so that people are supported on it. If there is not enough air in the lilo, it can bottom out, which is very uncomfortable and could cause pressure areas in people who are at risk.

Aims for using the equipment

- To provide movement stimulation.
- To provide tactile stimulation – the feel of the mat or covers on the bed/chair.
- To use as a prop in a sensory theme.
- For relaxation.
- Depending on how a person is moved on the water bed/lilo, this can be relaxing or stimulating. Slow movements are relaxing; faster movements are more stimulating.
- To provide an object of interest to promote communication – for example, encourage people to give eye contact to indicate 'more' before rocking the water bed/lilo again. This also teaches cause and effect because people learn that, when they look at you, the equipment will be moved again.

How to use the equipment to stimulate the different senses

Touch

- Sit the person in the chair/bed and feel the water moving beneath the cover.
- Lay the person on the lilo. Feel the vinyl or velour.

Copyright © Scope (Vic.) Ltd 2008

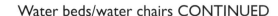

Movement

- Gently move the person on the bed/lilo.
- As the person moves themselves, they will experience different sensations as the water/air moves under them.

Seeing

- Not applicable

Hearing

- Not applicable

Smell

- Not applicable – unless giving a person a relaxing hand massage on the water bed using scented oils or lotions.

Other ways to use the equipment

- Make up different textured mats to put on the water bed.
- Use a black sheet and put the fibre-optic spray on it so that it contrasts with the background.
- Place fluorescent items on the black sheet and view under the UV light.

Cheaper and everyday alternatives

- Buy a lilo/air mattress. Although these are filled with air rather than water, they can produce a similar effect. They can be bought from camping shops and general stores. They are often velour on one side and vinyl on the other, which is easy to wipe down and keep clean. Mattress protectors and black or white fitted sheets are also useful to provide a contrasting background for other equipment. Buy a pump to help inflate the lilo.
- Put water or air in wine bladders. Feel the water or air move with hands or feet. These bags can also be decorated with fluorescent strips that glow under UV light, or covers can be made of different materials. Make pillow covers with Velcro® fastenings to go over the wine bladders. These can easily be removed for washing. Some fabrics – for example, black and white strips of material – show up well under UV light (see Figures 5.11 and 5.12 pp.127–8).
- There are some large, clear wine bladders available. These can be filled with water and white or fluorescent strips that show up well under UV light.
- Make gel bags by putting scented hair gel in resealable freezer bags or lock zip bags. Double bag the gel to keep the contents inside. These can be felt with hands or feet and some of the scent will seep through the bags.

Copyright © Scope (Vic.) Ltd 2008

Activities
SEEING

FIBRE-OPTIC SPRAYS

Description

The fibre-optic spray consists of a motor with light and colour wheel inside a box (light source) and 1.5, 2 or 3 metre long fibre-optic sprays coming out of the box. The fibre-optic spray usually has 200 or 300 strands of fibre optics. Each strand is composed of a plastic sleeve containing about 100 or 150 glass fibres inside. The fibre-optic sprays change colour as the colour wheel rotates, and some appear to flicker as the light passes through a blue and white-stripped portion of the colour wheel. The optical fibres are safe to touch, because there is no heat and no electricity in the strands. Plastic fibre optics can now be purchased through some companies. Instead of having 140 glass fibres, they have three strands of plastic down the sheathing (personal communications with Richard Hirstwood).

Sometimes the ends of the fibres are not glowing. This may be because too many of the glass strands have been broken along the length of the fibre and consequently the light is not conducted to the end of the fibre. There's not much that can be done about this, except cut the fibre where the light ends so that the light shines out of a shorter fibre. Remember to turn off the power when cutting the broken strands. The ends of the cut strands will need to be resealed. Extra caps for the ends of strands are available from the suppliers of the fibre-optic sprays. Contact the suppliers for further details before attempting repairs.

Fibre optics are also available as shimmering curtains, cascade fountains and fibre-optic carpets. The latter is when only the end of the fibre optic is seen as a tiny spot of light set into black or dark blue carpet. The spots of light are either set in a random pattern or specific shapes – for example, a star or concentric circle. The fibre-optic carpets can be used as walls, floors or ceilings. They are particularly effective if they are built into small, dark cubbyholes and used as the ceiling. People can then lie inside and look at the 'stars' in the sky. Interactive carpets are also available, which are operated through pressure either by pressing down with hands, walking over or rolling on. When pressure is applied, the lights change colour.

PRECAUTIONS

- The fibre optics need to be checked on a regular basis to ensure that none of them are broken or that the ends have split open; otherwise, the glass fibres inside the plastic sleeve may protrude. These could potentially break off and tiny particles of glass could be accidentally rubbed into eyes or skin. The individual glass fibres are very thin, so they may not be seen. However, sometimes people feel itchy as the tiny fibres get onto their skin.

Copyright © Scope (Vic.) Ltd 2008

- Some of the fibre optics have tiny caps on the end of each strand. If these come off, new caps can be glued back on. These are available from the manufacturer who sells the fibre-optic spray.

- The fibre optics should not be chewed because people can bite through the plastic sleeve and chew on the glass fibres.

- Be aware that the fibres can become tangled and need 'combing out' from time to time to untangle them.

- Do not cover the box containing the light source because it can overheat.

- Do not put the light source on soft play mats because it may stop the air flow to the light source unit and cause it to overheat.

- The box with the light source carries electricity. Ensure people keep away from this part and only interact with the fibre-optic strands.

- If the light source is fixed to the wall, make sure it is secure and cannot be pulled down. Also make sure that it can take the weight of the fibres hanging down.

- Do not tie the fibres in knots because this can break the glass strands. If all the strands inside a particular plastic sheath are broken, the light will not shine through to the end.

- Some people may associate the lights with heat and become anxious if the fibres are draped around them. First use the fibres on yourself to show that they are not harmful.

- People may need to be taught that not all lights are safe to touch.

- Talk with suppliers about how to change the globe/light bulb. Remember to disconnect the fibre-optic spray from the mains and let the globe cool down before touching it. Do not touch the glass section of the new globe with bare fingers because this can significantly reduce the life of the globe.

Copyright © Scope (Vic.) Ltd 2008

Aims for using the equipment

- For relaxation – it can be used with other equipment (e.g. quiet music to set up an environment for relaxation).
- To gain a person's attention.
- To provide visual stimulation and visual tracking (if the fibre optics are moved for visual tracking, remember to move them slowly; otherwise, people will not be able to track the fibres).
- To provide tactile stimulation; people can hold the fibres, feel them brushed on their face or hands, or be wrapped in them.
- To motivate people to hold objects.
- For switch practice if the fibre-optic spray is plugged into a power box.
- To teach cognitive skills – for example, colours, up/down, in front/behind (move the fibres into the different positions).

How to use the equipment to stimulate the different senses

Touch

- Feel the strands of fibre optics.
- Drape fibre optics around shoulders, limbs, hands. Do people dislike feeling fibre optics on certain parts of their bodies?

Movement

- Hold the fibres in different positions to encourage people to move their arms and reach out.

Seeing

- Watch fibre optics at a distance or close up. Do people notice the effects from afar? Are people more interested when the visual effects are near them?
- If the whole effect is too overpowering for someone, offer one strand at a time to look at.
- Vary the number of strands offered for people to look at.
- Observe a person's reactions to the fibre optics. Do they indicate a like or dislike for a particular colour?

Hearing

- Do people react to the gentle rustle of the fibres as they are shaken?

Smell

- Not applicable

Copyright © Scope (Vic.) Ltd 2008

Other ways to use the equipment

- Paint an old bicycle or wheelchair wheel white. Suspend it from the ceiling. Mount the light source box near the ceiling. Suspend the fibre optics from the wheel and let the ends drop down to form a shimmering circular curtain in which people can sit. Attach the fibre optics to a power box (see Figure 5.6) so that people can turn the fibre optics on when they like (Yooralla Glenroy).

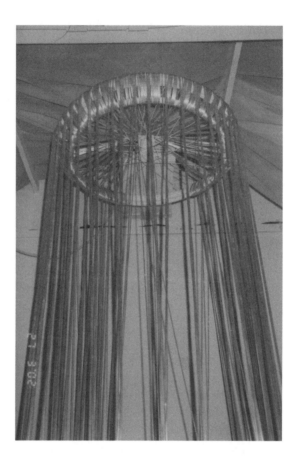

Figure 5.6 Fibre optics

- Thread the fibres through hoops, colanders and poles to create curtains and waterfalls (Richard Hirstwood).
- If a person is wearing thin clothing, push some of the fibres up their sleeve so that they can see the light moving on their body as well as feel it (Richard Hirstwood).
- Punch small holes in the top of a box and thread the fibres through to create a personal environment (Richard Hirstwood).
- Create another mini-environment by draping the fibres over a leaf chair. To make the environment even more enclosed, first drape a mosquito net or some lace over the leaf chair and then place the fibre optics around this.
- Mount the light source securely; then hang a net across the ceiling and lay the fibre-optics over it so you have a fibre optic ceiling effect (Richard Hirstwood).

 Copyright © Scope (Vic.) Ltd 2008

- Lay the fibres on a white mat and a black mat. See if people respond differently to the different backgrounds.
- The fibres can be draped around body parts for further tactile stimulation.
- The fibre-optic spray can be plugged into a power box to make it switch controlled.
- Use a mat switch so that people can roll on the mat to turn on the fibre optics, rather than having to use their hands.
- Ask someone to lie on the fibre optics, and put a pressure mat switch underneath so that they must roll on or off it to make it light up (Richard Hirstwood).
- Build a small trolley on wheels to house the fibre-optic spray. Make a top shelf to store the fibres and ensure that there is plenty of ventilation to the motor unit. The whole unit can easily be moved on the wheeled trolley so that the equipment can be used in other locations.

Cheaper and everyday alternatives

- Buy hand-held, battery-operated fibre-optic torches.
- Make holes in a box and insert the handles of six or more hand-held fibre-optic sprays to create a small fibre-optic 'bush'.
- Buy a fibre-optic lamp.
- Go to a fireworks display.
- Visit the Christmas displays.
- Visit a jewellery counter; buy glittery jewellery.

Copyright © Scope (Vic.) Ltd 2008

BUBBLE TUBES

Description

These are vertical Perspex™ tubes containing water. They are mounted to a base that contains a pump, light and colour wheel. The pump creates tiny bubbles that float up the clear perspex tube and, as the colour wheel rotates, it seems to make the bubbles change colour. A variation on the basic bubble tube is one that has a small central vertical tube and coloured balls. These balls are blown up through the central tube and float down around the outside of the tube.

Interactive bubble tubes are also available. These allow people to turn on the bubbles or lights. Switches can be colour codes so that they correspond with the colour of the bubbles inside the tube. For example, when the green switch is pressed, green bubbles float up the bubble tube. Some bubble tubes also have different configurations of bubbles so that, when a switch is pressed, either a single stream of bubbles or a mass of bubbles float up the tube.

PRECAUTIONS

- Remember to change the water in the bubble tubes regularly. Richard Hirstwood (in *A Practical Guide to the Use of Multisensory Rooms*) states that the British Water Authority advises that the water should be changed every six weeks. Other suppliers have recommended that the water should be changed when the bubble tubes are left unused for long periods of time – for example, over holidays. They also recommend that the water should be treated using a Milton tablet. Small pumps, which can be attached to a drill, can be used to empty the bubble tubes. Check with the supplier on how to empty and clean the bubble tube.

- Ensure that the bubble columns are safely attached to the wall; otherwise, they can be pulled over.

- Do not use paper towel to clean the tube or mirrors because it is abrasive and will scratch the plastic. Clean them using a soft cloth and a plastic safe cleaner. Some companies recommend the use of Mr Sheen™ as this has the added advantage of being anti-static, which helps repel dust.

- When changing the halogen globe, do not touch the globe with your fingers because the grease from your fingers can damage it.

Copyright © Scope (Vic.) Ltd 2008

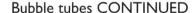

Aims for using the equipment

- To gain a person's attention.
- To provide visual and tactile/movement (vibration) stimulation.
- To create a relaxing environment.
- To encourage visual tracking (watching the bubbles).
- To practise switching skills.
- To teach cognitive skills (e.g. colours, up/down, stop/go).

How to use the equipment to stimulate the different senses

Touch

- Place hands around the tubes and feel the vibrations.
- Lie on mats next to the tubes and feel the vibrations.
- Feel the cool, smooth surface of the Perspex™.

Movement

- Encourage people to reach out to use the switch to start the bubble tube. Hold the switch in different positions to encourage reaching.
- Track bubbles with fingers on the tube.

Seeing

- Watch the coloured bubbles moving up the tube.
- Add plastic fish to the tubes and watch them bobbing in the water.
- Some bubble tubes have an inner central tube so watch the balls moving up and down in the water.
- Bubble tubes are often surrounded by mirrors to give the impression of multiple tubes. Are people more interested in looking at their reflections than the bubbles? Are people visually overwhelmed by the reflections of the bubble tubes(s)?

Hearing

- Are people distracted by the quiet hum of the bubble tube, or do they enjoy it? Where possible, have seating built around the bubble tube. People can then hug the tube and listen to the sound of the pump and the gurgles from the bubbles moving within the tube.

Smell

- Not applicable – unless the tube is part of a sea theme and there is seaweed nearby to smell.

Copyright © Scope (Vic.) Ltd 2008

Other ways to use the equipment

- Use the bubble tubes as a focus point when setting up the room for relaxation. Most people find the gentle flow of the coloured bubbles hypnotizing. Add relaxing music, dimmed lighting and soothing oils to create a multisensory environment for relaxation.

- Purchase an interactive bubble tube so that people can practise switching skills and learn cause and effect.

- Position people different distances from the bubble tube. Do they need to be close to them to notice that they are there?

- Test reaction to sound. Turn people away so they cannot see the bubble tube; do they react when the pump is turned on?

- Use in a story/production (e.g. *Moby Dick, Jonah and the Whale*).

- Use as a setting to recount an outing (e.g. visit to the aquarium).

- Set up a game, with different people in charge of the different coloured switches. Call out a colour so that the person holding that coloured switch can operate it to change the colours in the bubble tube (ensure that the bubble tube has this option, whereby pressing a certain coloured switch results in the corresponding coloured bubbles in the tube).

- Build a seat/plinth around the base of the bubble tube so that people can get close to the tube and hug or lie next to it to feel the vibrations.

Cheaper and everyday alternatives

- Small bubble tubes are available from general commercial outlets. Some run on 240v electricity so check that they are safe. The large bubble columns usually have a transformer in them to reduce the power outlet.

- Put gel in ziplock plastic bags, add paint/food dye and move the bags with your hands.

- Make bubble mix and use a variety of wands (including giant wands) to blow bubbles.

- Put bubble bath in a footspa and watch the bubbles foam up.

- Put bubble bath in the bath.

- Use a blender to make foamy coffee or milo.

    Copyright © Scope (Vic.) Ltd 2008

HURRICANE TUBES WITH MIRRORS

Description

These are two-metre vertical Perspex™ tubes mounted to a base. Inside the base, there is a pump for air and a halogen lamp. The tube contains small, lightweight balls and mirrors are either mounted to the base or attached to the walls around the tube. They are similar to the bubble tubes but contain air instead of water.

The mirrors enhance the visual effect provided by the balls moving in the air column. Some people find the ball movement motivating to watch. Others are not interested in the balls themselves, but are more motivated by the shadows moving on the ceiling. Other people are aroused or motivated by the noise, while some enjoy the vibrations felt through the tube. It is a good piece of equipment to alert people rather than for relaxation.

The hurricane tube has the equivalent to a power box built into the base to make it switch interactive. People can control the air, and hence the balls moving in the tube, via a switch. The switch control can be set to 'momentary', so the balls only move when the switch is continually pressed, 'latched', where the switch needs to be pressed to start and stop the balls, and 'timed'. With the 'timed' element, when the switch is pressed, the balls move for a predetermined time and stop. People then have to operate the switch again to set the balls moving. If the balls move all the time, then people may have no incentive to use the switch. If the balls move continually, the sensory stimulation can lose its effect as people cease to notice the moving balls.

PRECAUTIONS

- Be aware that the flickering of the hurricane tube may cause some people to have seizures.

- When the globe needs to be replaced, unscrew the base and carefully remove the old globe. When inserting the new halogen globe, be careful not to touch the front of it with fingers as the grease from fingers can damage it.

Aims for using the equipment

- To arouse and alert.
- To gain a person's visual and auditory attention (seeing and hearing).
- To provide visual, auditory (hearing) and tactile/movement (vibration) stimulation
- To provide the opportunity for visual tracking.
- To practise switching skills.
- To teach cognitive skills (e.g. colours, up/down, stop/go).

How to use the equipment to stimulate the different senses

Touch

- Place hands on the air column or base to feel the vibrations. Hug the column to feel the vibrations through the body.

Movement

- Encourage people to reach out to use the switch to start the hurricane tube. Hold the switch in different positions to encourage reaching.

Seeing

- Watch different coloured and tinsel balls being blown around in the air column.
- Watch the shadows created on the ceiling.
- Look for the switch.

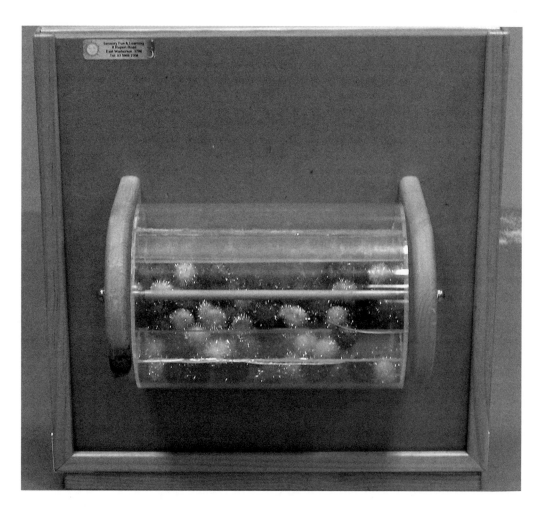

Figure 5.7 Glitter roll

  Copyright © Scope (Vic.) Ltd 2008

Hearing

- Listen to the sound of the pump as it blows the balls through the air column.

Smell

- Not applicable.

Cheaper and everyday alternatives

- Toys with a fan and glitter pom poms. These are available as switch-operated toys so that, when a switch is pressed, the fan comes on and the pom poms fly around inside a Perspex™ dome.
- Equipment with Perspex™ rolls and glitter pom poms inside (see Figure 5.7).
- Use a fan and attach different pieces of material to the grille as streamers. Activate the fan using a power box and switch.
- Dress up using glitter wigs and glasses, and look in the mirror.

Copyright © Scope (Vic.) Ltd 2008

PHOTO SOLAR PROJECTOR

Description

The photo solar projector is a light unit that is used with cassettes or wheels to project images onto different surfaces. Effects wheels are either liquid wheels or theme wheels. The liquid wheels are made of coloured liquids, which become more fluid as they are heated up by the lamp from the projector. These colours then move and merge into each other creating interesting visual effects. There are a variety of theme effects wheels – for example, balloons, undersea and fireworks.

There are a number of extra lenses that can be purchased for the photo solar projector. They create different images by splitting images, deflecting images and rotating them in different ways. Some people may find this interesting, but others can find it visually over-simulating and confusing.

There are a number of disadvantages with the solar projector:

- Many of the theme wheels are visually busy with too many pictures and objects placed close to each other. This may be visually over-stimulating and, for people who can identify pictures, there may be too much detail for them to identify the different images.

- The wheel rotates in a circular fashion that is difficult for some people to track.

- As the wheel rotates, partial pictures emerge, which some people may find difficult to identify.

Despite the disadvantages, one of the best features of the solar effects projector is the ability to make and customize effects wheels. This means including as much or as little detail on the wheels as required. The wheels can also be individualized and include people, places and things that have meaning to people looking at the projections.

To make effects wheels, print out photographs or clip art onto acetate and put these within a blank effects wheel. Coloured gel (that look like thick cellophane used over lights by disco companies) can also be used. Instructions on how to make effects wheels are available in Appendix 10. Richard Hirstwood also has a website giving detailed instructions on how to make your own wheels – www.multi-sensory-room.co.uk (go to 'sensory ideas' and select 'making wheels').

PRECAUTIONS

- Keep people away from the projector unit because it becomes hot.

- Always have a wheel in the gate; otherwise, the plastic parts of the lens assembly can melt.

- Always have the wheel rotating; otherwise, the wheel can be damaged.

- Ensure that there is air circulating around the unit; otherwise, it can overheat.

- Some manufacturers say not to tip the projector at a steep angle because it can shorten the life of the globe.

- Remember to turn off the unit at the mains when changing the globe.

 Copyright © Scope (Vic.) Ltd 2008

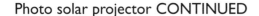

- When changing the globe, remember not to handle it. Open the plastic covering from the bottom to expose the metal prongs and push it into place while holding the top of the globe within its plastic cover.

- Remember to wait for the old globe to cool down before trying to remove it.

- If using the projector on a shelf, remember to ensure that it is safely secured and that there is a power socket at shelf height. This eliminates trailing wires and extension cords because these are a potential safety hazard.

- Do not use with a switching system because constantly turning the unit on and off can blow the globe or fuse.

- When focusing the lens, be careful not to rotate it too far anti-clockwise because it can come all the way out and drop to the ground.

Aims for using the equipment

- For relaxation – it can be used with other equipment (e.g. quiet music to set up an environment for relaxation); use a liquid wheel.
- To gain a person's attention.
- To provide visual stimulation and visual tracking (watching the pictures rotate).
- To use as a visual aid to a story or theme.
- To use as a visual aid to teach a task.
- To use to display people's art work.
- To teach cognitive skills (e.g. colours, picture recognition).
- To use as a topic of conversation – take pictures of an outing people have been on.
- To provide visual stimulation.

How to use the equipment to stimulate the different senses

Touch

- Not applicable.

Movement

- Not applicable.

Copyright © Scope (Vic.) Ltd 2008

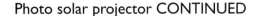

Seeing

- Watch the different colours, patterns and pictures moving around the room.

Hearing

- Not applicable.

Smell

- Not applicable.

Other ways to use the equipment

- Use clip art or take photos of people. Scan the images into the computer and use them to design an effects wheel. If the colours appear washed out, print out two acetates of the same picture and put them both in the effects wheel to get a denser coloured picture.

- Take photographs of trips and make into a wheel to project onto the wall. Use this as a talking point when remembering the outing. People who require sensory-focused activities may be interested in watching the moving colours without recognizing the images.

- Scan photos of people doing different parts of a task in order to teach them the sequence of that task. Remember to follow this with a practical session where people get to do the task.

- Cut up pieces of coloured gel (used over spotlights in discos) and create patterns in the blank wheel.

- Make up a wheel to complement a story (e.g. *The Hungry Caterpillar).*

- Make up a wheel to complement a theme (e.g. make up a wheel of boats and windsurfers to project in a beach theme).

- Draw directly onto acetate and project these pictures.

- Stick slide photos of places/people onto the wheels.

- People can create drawings on the computer that can then be printed onto acetate and projected onto the wall as an art show.

- The solar effects wheels can be used to project images onto a wall, or onto different surfaces – for example, lace curtain, mosquito netting, survival blanket, holographic paper – to get different effects. Material such as lace can be hung in a curtain and used as a projection screen, or crumpled in a heap to give a 3D effect.

- Make up a projection screen using a sheet of white Lycra®.

- Make kites out of light coloured material to project on to (Richard Hirstwood).

- Shine the projector into a box lined with hologram wrapping paper or survival blanket (Richard Hirstwood).

- Project images from the projector onto a white umbrella. People can look at the image from a distance, or sit under the umbrella for a different experience.

Copyright © Scope (Vic.) Ltd 2008

Cheaper and everyday alternatives

- If looking for visual stimulation, think about torches. Coloured cellophane can be placed over torches for different effects. Torches with plastic covers, which can be clipped over the front to create different patterns and colours, can also be bought.

- To create an interesting visual effect, make pinprick holes in a piece of card and shine a torch through it onto a wall.

- Make holes in a piece of card and cover the back with dark blue cellophane. Shine a torch through it onto the ceiling to create a starry sky.

- Shine a torch onto glittery material (e.g. holographic paper, mirror tiles, car sun shade).

- Use a slide projector or overhead projector (OHP).

Copyright © Scope (Vic.) Ltd 2008

SLIDE PROJECTORS

Description

A slide projector can be used as an alternative to the solar projector. If purchasing a slide projector, consider buying the box ones with a slide carousel on top. These can be used to project images onto surfaces, but they also have a small TV screen so that people can look at the images close up. Also check that this type of slide projector has a cassette unit with it. This means that sound effects or a narrative can be added to go with the slides. The slide projector is gradually being replaced by data projectors used with a computer.

The other advantage of the slide projector is that it can be switch adapted. This means that people can be in control of changing the slides.

PRECAUTIONS

- Take note of where people are sitting in order to ensure that the light from the projector does not shine into their eyes.

Aims for using the equipment

- For relaxation – it can be used with other equipment (e.g. quiet music to set up an environment for relaxation); project images of flowers and trees.
- To gain a person's attention.
- To provide visual stimulation and visual tracking (by moving a slide projector located on a table with wheels).
- For switch practice if the slide projector is switch adapted.
- To use as a visual aid to a story or theme.
- To use as a visual aid to teach a task.
- To use to display people's art work.
- To teach cognitive skills (e.g. colours, picture recognition).
- To use as a topic of conversation – take pictures of an outing people have been on.

How to use the equipment to stimulate the different senses

Touch

- Not applicable – unless the projector is switch adapted and used with a textured switch.

Movement

- Encourage people to reach out to the switch to change the slides.

Copyright © Scope (Vic.) Ltd 2008

Seeing

- Watch the different colours, patterns and pictures projected onto different surfaces.

Hearing

- Play relaxing music on the cassette portion of the slide projector while projecting soothing images.

Smell

- Not applicable

Other ways to use the equipment

- Project different images onto the wall for people to look at. Some people may find it easier to locate and look at stationary pictures, rather than the moving ones created by the solar projector. Some people may also be cued to look when they hear the slide change.
- To create moving images, project pictures onto a lace curtain or strips of white cloth, which are gently moved by the wind from the fan.
- Sit in a leaf chair and drape netting over the frame. Project images onto this.
- Project images onto a wall, or onto different surfaces – for example, lace curtain, mosquito netting, survival blanket, holographic paper – to get different effects. The lace etc. can be hung in a curtain and used as a projection screen, or crumpled in a heap to give a 3D effect.
- Project images onto a small beach tent.
- A large piece of white Lycra® makes an effective projection screen. Fasten it onto hooks from the ceiling and attach it to heavy sand bags on the floor (Helen Dilkes).
- Place the slide projector on a table with wheels. This way, the images can be slowly moved around the room to practise visual tracking.
- Take pictures of real objects that have meaning for people, and use those for picture identification sessions.
- Take slides of different people to practise person identification skills.
- Make up theme slides and use outings to take pictures for these themes (e.g. shops and signs, people we know, numbers and colours, the environment). Slides of graffiti provide interesting shapes and colours for another theme (Helen Dilkes). To make it more motivating for people, take photos of them as well. For example, if the theme is nature, take photos of people at the beach, eating ice-cream or walking in the park, as well as the seagulls, water, sand, trees, flowers, etc.
- Use slides for colour/number recognition work.
- Use the slides as a prompt for discussion (e.g. of different themes, places you have visited, who went on the trip).

Copyright © Scope (Vic.) Ltd 2008

- Use the slide projector to present a show that documents a person's life or an important event in their life. Take slides of different activities, places, objects or people that are important to a person. Record commentaries onto the cassette tape and encourage people to change the slides by using a switch. They can then be in control of sharing important things in their lives with other people.
- Take photos of art work and have an art show.
- Take slides of relaxing images (e.g. streams, woodland) and use with the cassette part to create a relaxing environment.
- Take slides and recordings of everyday sounds (e.g. a bus, birds, a telephone, or an individual's vocalizations or speech).
- Make up fluorescent collages and take slide pictures of them under UV light. Slides of deep space themes with different stars, planets and white clouds, which are projected in the multisensory room, are very effective. Images can be projected onto a wall or lace curtains. Create the illusion of movement by using a fan to move the lace curtain as images are projected onto it.
- Create slides by reusing old slides that are no longer needed. Bleach them to remove the old picture but make sure that the plastic framed slides, not the paper ones, are used, because the latter will disintegrate in the bleach. Rinse the slides well. Alternatively, blank slides are available from some photographic shops.
- To create your own picture, use different types of pens, coloured paints with a dense colour or gel paints. Make sure that the paints used don't melt in the slide projector. Some felt pens project a very washed-out effect.
- To produce a different effect, scratch the slide film with sand paper and colour with felt pens.
- Take slide film of boards made up with fluorescent/white paints, fluorescent/white objects and photograph under UV light.
- Buy packages of different themes of slides – for example, 'Galaxies' packs that have pictures of different planets. These are sometimes available from science museums.
- Use slides to teach a sequence, which can also be followed up in another session (e.g. learning the sequence to turn the tape-recorder on).

Copyright © Scope (Vic.) Ltd 2008

OVERHEAD PROJECTORS

Description

Overhead projectors (OHPs) are not widely used these days because computers and data projectors have replaced them. They consist of a light source and a box so that information on transparencies can be projected onto a wall. They offer a cheaper way to project images than the solar projector.

> **PRECAUTION**
>
> - Take note of where people are sitting in order to ensure that the light from the projector does not shine into their eyes.

Aims for using the equipment

- For relaxation – it can be used with other equipment (e.g. quiet music to set up an environment for relaxation); project images of flowers and trees and soothing coloured shapes.
- To gain a person's attention.
- To provide visual stimulation and visual tracking (by moving the projector on a table with wheels).
- To use as a visual aid to a story or theme.
- To use as a visual aid to teach a task.
- To use to display people's art work.
- To teach cognitive skills (e.g. colours, picture recognition).
- To use as a topic of conversation – take pictures of an outing people have been on.

How to use the equipment to stimulate the different senses

Touch

- Not applicable.

Movement

- Not applicable.

Seeing

- Watch the different colours, patterns and pictures projected onto different surfaces.

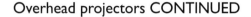

Hearing

- Not applicable.

Smell

- Not applicable.

Other ways to use the equipment

- Project a beam of light by cutting a circle in a piece of paper and putting it on the OHP. Alternatively, use the inner sleeve of a record cover. Place the OHP on a small trolley and move the trolley so that people can visually follow the spot of light as it moves across the wall or screen.

- Create a night scene by cutting out stars and make small holes in a piece of paper with a knitting needle or pin. Try making holes in blue acetate for a blue sky with stars.

- Create a stained-glass effect by cutting patterns out of a piece of paper and covering the holes with coloured tissue paper/cellophane or sweet wrappers (use those made from cellophane and you have the excuse of eating the sweets!).

- Use different coloured acetates with shapes cut out of them, and put objects on the acetates.

- Objects to use on the acetate:
  - coloured lens covers for swimming pool lights
  - foil sweet papers
  - translucent glass beads (they're used to keep flowers in place in vases).

- When using objects, put acetate down first so that the glass on the OHP is not scratched. Objects may also be spun on the acetate.

- Draw on acetates with coloured pens/paints.

- Put coloured cellophane on the acetates in a variety of patterns.

- Put a Pyrex® bowl filled with water or oil on the OHP and drip inks into it. (Try doing marbling on the OHP.) N.B. Only use water on the OHP if your OHP is one of the portable ones that has the electrical components at the back, in order to prevent any water placed on the glass coming into contact with the electrical parts.

- To create movement with the visual projections, place the OHP on a small table with castors that can be easily moved.

- Judy Denziloe presented the above ideas at a multi-sensory environments conference in the UK in October 1997.

- Make up a cardboard overlay with cut-out shapes. Put coloured cellophane over the shapes and project them onto a mirror ball. The colours will then be projected around the room by the rotating mirror ball.

- Print out photos and pictures onto coloured acetate to use in a sensory story or with a specific topic of conversation.

 Copyright © Scope (Vic.) Ltd 2008

MIRROR BALLS, SPOTLIGHTS AND COLOUR WHEELS

Description

These pieces of equipment are often used together. The mirror ball can be stationary or revolving. If using a revolving mirror ball, select the slowest one possible. Disco-type mirror balls revolve far too quickly and can over-stimulate people and make them feel sick. A spotlight is shone onto the mirror ball and through a revolving colour wheel. This gives the effect of spots of changing colour, which also revolve around the room if the mirror ball is moving.

Portable battery-operated mirror balls are also available, but the speed cannot be adjusted on these and they may move too quickly for some people. Mirror balls of different sizes that can be suspended, but do not rotate, can be purchased from many commercial outlets.

When having a mirror ball, spotlight and colour wheel installed, ask for the spotlight and colour wheel to be wired up so that a switch can be used to control them. If this isn't wired through an integrated switching system, run long cords from the ceiling in conduits. The plugs can then be put into power boxes/power links and the spotlight can then be turned on via a switch, even though the equipment is located on the ceiling. People can be in control of turning on the light and creating the coloured spots effect.

Think about where the mirror ball will be suspended, in its relationship to the spotlight and where the spotlight is projected onto the mirror ball, because these factors will give different effects. If the spotlight and the mirror ball are far apart, the spots from the mirror ball will spread out over the room, look larger and appear to travel faster. If the mirror ball and spotlight are located closer together, smaller spots of light will be created. The spots of light will appear to travel more slowly. The closer the mirror ball and spotlight are located, the smaller and more intense the spots appear because they only cover a small area.

Also think about where in the room the mirror ball will be suspended. If it is in the middle of the room, it will cast spots of light around the whole room. However, some people might not like the spots being projected onto them. It may be better to hang the mirror ball in the corner of a room. That way, people who love the spots can sit under the mirror ball and be bathed in lights. Others who can't tolerate that intensity of stimulation, but still like looking at the lights, can sit in the other corner and watch the lights without being surrounded by them. Experiment with the room, moving the mirror ball and spotlight to different locations and angling the spotlight onto different parts of the mirror ball. If the spotlight is directed onto the middle of the mirror ball reflections will appear all around the room. Only half the room will be covered by the spots of light if the spotlight is shone onto the side of the mirror ball.

Some people cannot tolerate the moving lights created by the revolving mirror ball. It is advisable that, when a person first enters the multisensory room, the mirror ball should be stationary. Once people become accustomed to the room, start the mirror ball revolving and observe closely for any adverse reactions.

Copyright © Scope (Vic.) Ltd 2008

PRECAUTIONS

- Observe for any signs of agitation or sickness when the mirror ball is revolving.

- Initially use the mirror ball without it rotating. Check how people respond to the lights, and then set the mirror ball rotating. Observe very carefully because some people may feel sick with the spinning lights. If people appear distressed, turn it off immediately.

- Ensure that the ceiling can take the weight of the mirror ball.

Aims for using the equipment

- For visual stimulation.
- For visual tracking.
- To motivate people to attend.
- To teach the concept of on/off (when used with a switch).
- To teach the concept of cause and effect.
- To practise switching skills.
- To help create a relaxing environment.

How to use the equipment to stimulate the different senses

Touch

- If creating a home-made 'mirror ball', encourage people to help by being involved in the papier mâché process. Feel the finished mirror ball.

Movement

- Encourage people to reach out and use a switch.
- If using a papier mâché mirror ball, suspend it low enough that people can reach out to knock it.

Seeing

- Watch stationary spots of coloured light.
- Watch different coloured spots of light moving slowly around the room.

Hearing

- Not applicable.

Copyright © Scope (Vic.) Ltd 2008

Smell

- Not applicable.

Other ways to use the equipment

- Use a beach tent as an individual sensory environment. Suspend a small mirror ball from a piece of tape sewn onto the tent. Darken the tent with additional material over it if needed. Shine a torch onto the mirror ball to create dots of light. To make the environment interactive, attach a lamp to a power box and direct it onto the mirror ball. Encourage people to use a switch to turn the light on.

- Use the mirror ball as part of a theme environment (e.g. disco, planets).

- Use the mini sensory environment as part of a 'caves' theme.

- Shine the projector onto the mirror ball instead of the spotlight.

- Make overlays for the overhead projector with cut-outs covered with coloured cellophane. Direct the beam onto the mirror ball for a different effect (see Figure 5.8).

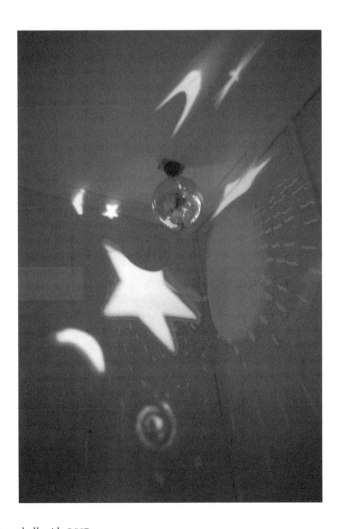

Figure 5.8 Mirror ball with OHP

Copyright © Scope (Vic.) Ltd 2008

Cheaper and everyday alternatives

- Make your own mirror ball. Decorate a papier mâché balloon with mirror tiles, or make up a cloth cover for a balloon, covered in mirror tile material or material with sequins (see Figure 5.9). Directing a fan onto the balloon can produce the effect of movement. The fan can be connected to a power box so that people are in control of moving the 'mirror ball'.

- Make up a mirror board with mirror, shiny buttons, tinfoil, etc.

- Buy small mirror balls, suspend and shine a torch on them.

- Look at your reflection in a mirror. Cover the mirror with shaving foam and wipe it away to reveal your face.

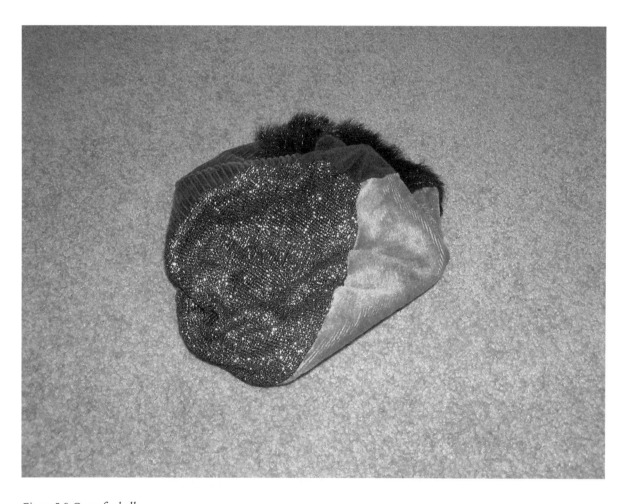

Figure 5.9 Cover for ball

 Copyright © Scope (Vic.) Ltd 2008

MAGIC LIGHTS/ROPE LIGHTS

Description

These are a rope of individual lights encased in a plastic tube. The lights travel along the tube at various speeds, sometimes staying on rather than moving and sometimes fading in and out. This piece of equipment can be plugged into a power box so that people can control it via a switch.

PRECAUTIONS

- On the fast speeds, the rope lights can cause people to have seizures due to the strobe effect.

- Be careful using the flashing bulbs on the fairy lights as they could cause a seizure.

- Ensure that you buy low voltage lights.

- Constant bending of the tube will break the internal wires and bulbs, which are too expensive to repair.

- Take care when mounting the lights because the wires can look messy and also become a hazard that people can trip over or pull.

Aims for using the equipment

- To motivate people to look – visual attention.
- To provide visual stimulation.
- To encourage people to visually track (use on slow speeds).
- To practise switching skills.
- To teach the concept of cause and effect.
- To teach the concept of on/off.
- To provide tactile stimulation (holding the tube).
- To teach cognitive skills – for example, colours (when the lights are not flashing fast).
- To create a relaxing environment.

How to use the equipment to stimulate the different senses

Touch

- Feel the smooth plastic of the casing.

Movement

- Hold the rope lights out in different positions to encourage people to reach out and touch/hold.

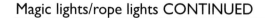

Seeing

- Watch the lights travelling along the tube.
- Watch the colours pulsing.
- Look at the different coloured lights.

Hearing

- Not applicable.

Smell

- Not applicable.

Other ways to use the equipment

- Plug the lights into a power box and encourage the people to use a switch to turn them on.
- Make up a tactile wall and incorporate the lights as part of the wall.

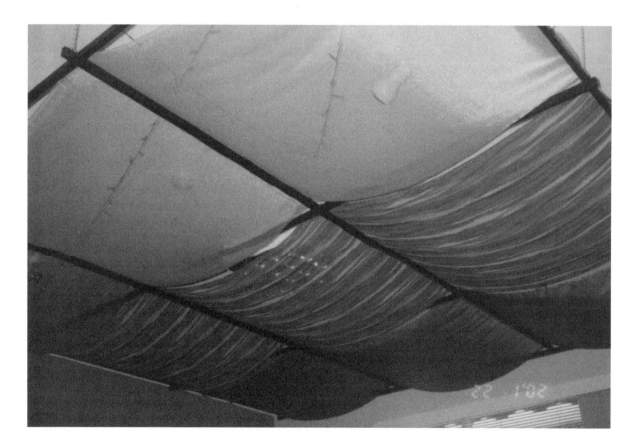

Figure 5.10 Lights above fabric

Copyright © Scope (Vic.) Ltd 2008

Cheaper and everyday alternatives

- Tree/fairy lights – these can be purchased from hardware stores. Some have stationary lights and others have moving or flashing ones. A strobe globe can replace one of the ordinary bulbs to give a flashing effect. These can also be purchased from hardware stores, but are difficult to buy other than at Christmas. Musical lights can also be purchased – for example, with Christmas carols.

- Use the fairy lights with other equipment (e.g. quiet music to set up an environment for relaxation). Take care not to have too many light sources on at the same time as it can be over-stimulating. Choose which ones you will use to create a relaxing environment.

- Suspend fairy lights from the ceiling and hang thin pieces of fabric beneath them. The lights will then shine through the fabric (see Figure 5.10)

- Sew lights behind a piece of black fabric to create a sparkling curtain.

- Hang fairy lights as a curtain with foil streamers.

- Make up a tactile wall and incorporate the fairy lights as part of the wall. Drill small holes into the wood and firmly attach the lights through the holes with the wiring behind the wall.

- Hand-held battery-operated torches can be purchased that have as an attachment a series of coloured lights encased in a plastic tube (similar to the rope lights).

Copyright © Scope (Vic.) Ltd 2008

ULTRA VIOLET (UV) LAMPS

Description

UV lamps have been used in dark rooms for a number of years. More recently they have been incorporated into multisensory rooms as a UV corner or corridor. Some rooms have been divided with thick curtains, white on one side and black on the other, so that one room can be divided into a white and dark room.

Another option is a portable UV cabinet. This is a small black box with a UV tube built into it. As it is portable, it can be used in different locations and be placed on a table for close-up work. However, some people may prefer the effect of being surrounded by darkness and seeing fluorescent objects in a larger area.

PRECAUTIONS

- Do not look directly into the light – angle the lamp down or build a pelmet around the UV light tube.

- Do not use after a massage with certain essential oils – for example, bergamot, which makes the skin more sensitive to UV and can cause a sunburn effect. Check with an aromatherapist before using essential oils.

- Some drugs will also make people more sensitive to the UV – check people's medication and precautions.

- There seems to be little consensus on what is considered safe. As a rule, only use the equipment for 30 minutes at a time or, if your eyes feel strained or you are getting a headache, have shorter sessions. Support people are more likely to be exposed to the UV for longer than the people with disabilities, especially if carrying out consecutive assessments.

- Flo Longhorn quotes research from Dr Brian Duffey who gives the example of 'a teacher and pupil working for two hours in a darkroom, approximately four feet (1.2 metres) from the light source. This would result in a dose of UV radiation equivalent to about 48 seconds of summer sunshine. He concludes that, if UV light is used appropriately in darkrooms, then there is no risk to the eyes or skin' (Longhorn 1997, p.5).

- When replacing a light tube, remember to use a blue-black one, which looks purple when it is turned off. Do not get the ones that look white because these are for sun beds. They do not cause objects to fluoresce and they are hazardous to use in a multisensory room.

- Be aware that some people may feel threatened or claustrophobic in dark spaces.

Copyright © Scope (Vic.) Ltd 2008

Aims for using the equipment

- To gain and maintain attention – some people are easily distracted by extraneous visual stimuli; in a dark room/area, objects can be presented one at a time and highlighted by the UV lamp, while other objects are hidden in the darkness.
- To provide visual stimulation.
- To encourage visual tracking – move objects manually or suspend them.
- To teach cognitive skills (e.g. colours, picture recognition, object recognition, numbers).
- To use as a visual aid to a story or theme.
- To use as a visual aid to teach a task.
- To use to display people's art work.

How to use the equipment to stimulate the different senses

Touch

- Provide different textured white and fluorescent objects for people to feel.

Movement

- Encourage people to reach out and touch the objects.
- Encourage people to reach out and use a fan with a power box and switch to make fluorescent and white objects move.

Seeing

- Look at the different colours glowing under the UV light.

Hearing

- Use fluorescent objects that also make a sound (e.g. fluorescent balls with bells inside).

Smell

- Add scent to fluorescent materials.

Other ways to use the equipment

- Make a portable UV lamp by using a table lamp and buying a small blue-black tube to put in it.
- Place fluorescent or white objects on a lilo covered with a black sheet. Move the lilo to make the objects bounce slightly or encourage people to move on the lilo to make the objects bounce.
- Make up a tactile wine bladder cover (as in Figure 5.11) using black and white or fluorescent materials. Fill the wine bladders with air or water for different effects. Make the covers like pillowslips that can be velcroed shut and easily removed for washing.

Copyright © Scope (Vic.) Ltd 2008

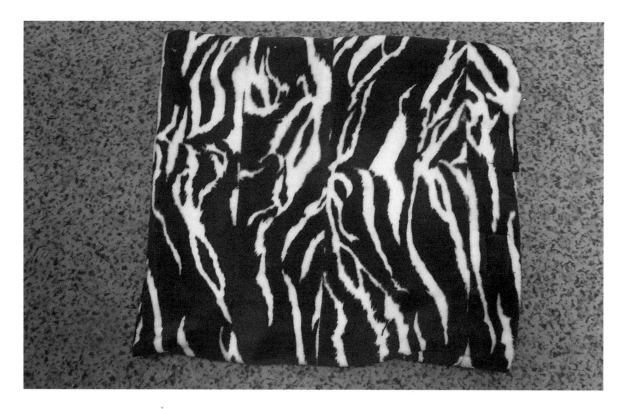

Figure 5.11: Wine bladder cover

- Stick strips of fluorescent paper onto an inflated wine bladder (see Figure 5.12).
- Make up balloon covers from white and fluorescent material. Suspend them and encourage people to reach out to make them move, or move them with the wind generated by a fan.
- Make up scenes using fluorescent paint, paper plates, napkins and other objects.
- Make a collage using white, glow-in-the-dark and other objects that show up under UV light (see Figure 5.13). Take a photograph/slide photo of the collage and project it in the multisensory room.
- Paint on black paper with fluorescent paints. Display in a UV light gallery.
- Paint on white tulle with fluorescent paint. Scrunch up into a heap and display as a 3D piece of art under UV light. Use large pieces of tulle and encourage people to 'paint' by rolling their wheelchairs over the material. Make sure water-based paints are used so that the wheelchairs can easily be cleaned.
- Highlight different objects with strips of fluorescent paper; draw with fluorescent pens and velcro on dots of fluorescent material.
- Make up/buy fluorescent dough to use under UV light using fluorescent cutters.
- Attach fluorescent or white material strips to a thick piece of dowel to make up streamer wands. People can shake the wand and watch the streamers move under the UV light. For people who have difficulty holding onto things, make a neoprene strap to keep the handles in the hand (see Figure 5.14).
- Some fishing line has a blue tinge to it – this glows well under UV light. Attach it to dowel handles to make wands. Fluorescent fishing line can also be purchased.

Copyright © Scope (Vic.) Ltd 2008

Ultra violet (UV) lamps CONTINUED

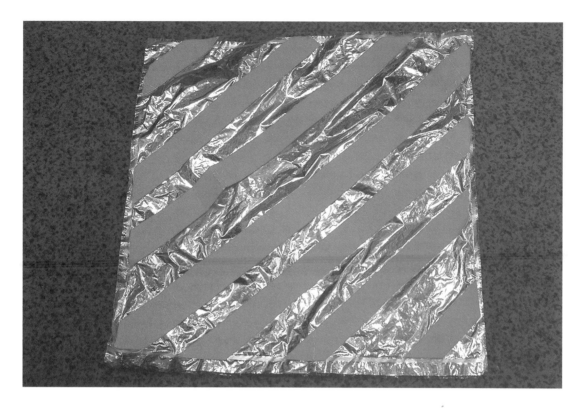

Figure 5.12: Fluorescent wine bladder

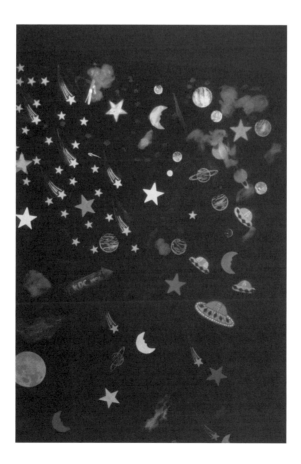

Figure 5.13 Collage under UV

- Stick strips of fluorescent ripstop nylon (parachute material) onto a hoop (see Figure 2.1 p.29). Suspend it under UV light and make the strips move by directing a fan onto the streamers.
- Work on body awareness by:
  - using white gloves to bring attention to people's hands
  - painting nails with fluorescent nail varnish
  - wearing fluorescent wigs
  - wearing fluorescent bands and bracelets
  - wearing fluorescent glass frames
  - using fluorescent sun block.
- Remember that the aim is for people to visually attend to objects in the natural environment and not just under UV light. As people are more able to attend to stimuli under UV light, start to present fluorescent objects with just a spotlight trained on them. Gradually increase the light in the room and offer fluorescing items in natural light without the spotlight.
- *Enhancing Education through the Use of Ultraviolet Light and Fluorescing Materials* – Flo Longhorn 1997 – is full of useful ideas.

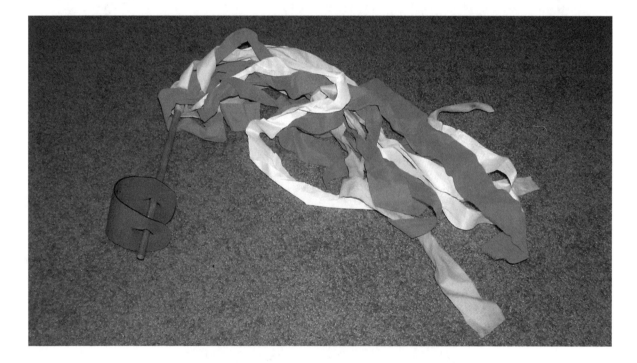

Figure 5.14 Neoprene strap on fluro wand

        Copyright © Scope (Vic.) Ltd 2008

INFINITY TUNNELS

Description

This is a box containing mirrors and lights. When turned on, the lights look as if they stretch on for ever. They do provide an interesting visual effect but, if this is all that the equipment does, then people could soon become bored. It is vital that equipment chosen can be used in many different ways so that it can meet not only people's current needs but also their changing needs. Some infinity tunnels are now interactive through the use of switches or sound activated so that the lights change in reaction to music or someone vocalizing.

PRECAUTIONS

- Be careful using the flashing lights with people who have epilepsy.

- Some people may become confused or disorientated looking at a never-ending row of lights.

Aims for using the equipment

- To gain people's attention.
- To provide visual stimulation.
- to teach cause and effect and practise switching skills.
- To learn about colours.
- As an aid to relaxation – some people may be mesmerized by watching the lights, which could help them to relax.

How to use the equipment to stimulate the different senses

Touch

- Not applicable – unless the switches have tactile surfaces.

Movement

- Encourage people to reach out to the switch to turn on the lights.

Seeing

- Watch the coloured lights moving and changing.
- Watch the lights change in response to a person's vocalizations.
- Position people to look into the lights and mirrors and set the unit on the timer. Encourage them to watch for the lights going off, then use their switch to turn them back on.

Hearing

- Listen to the music and watch the lights change in time to the music.

Copyright © Scope (Vic.) Ltd 2008

Smell

- Not applicable.

Other ways to use the equipment

Use as part of a group activity to promote hand–eye co-ordination, eye contact and to maintain attention. People are seated in a circle around the infinity tunnel and the leader sings 'Who who who is in the mirror?' The chosen person gets to activate the lights at the appropriate time (Lynda Anderson, occupational therapist).

Cheaper and everyday alternatives

- Cheaper versions of the infinity tunnel can be purchased from department stores. They measure 14 × 10 inches and create the same effect as the infinity tunnel. They can be made interactive by being turned on through a power box. Their small size means that they are portable and can be used in a multisensory room or other venues.
- Look at yourself in a mirror. Cover the mirror with shaving foam and wipe it away to reveal your image.
- Purchase a mirror covered with a metal bead curtain (see Figure 5.15)
- Use torches to shine onto reflective surfaces (e.g. holographic paper, tin foil, silver tinsel).

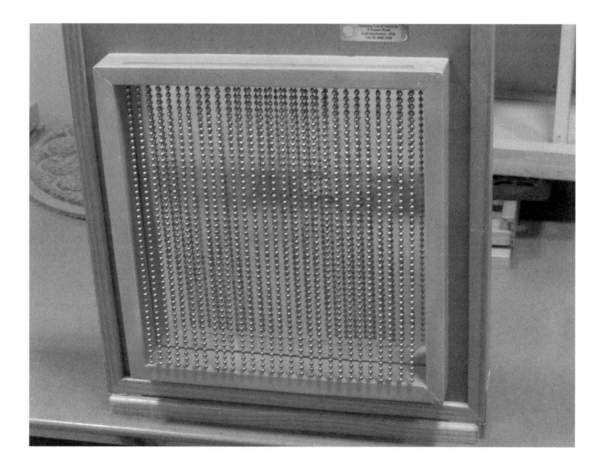

Figure 5.15 Mirror with metal curtain

 Copyright © Scope (Vic.) Ltd 2008

CATHERINE WHEELS

Description

These are light panels with spokes of small lights radiating out in a catherine wheel pattern. They are switch operated with push-button switches, or there are switch sockets so that different types of switches can be used to operate the lights display. There are a number of functions so that people can change the patterns and speeds of the lights. This is an expensive piece of equipment, so consider whether it does enough different things to justify the cost.

PRECAUTION

- Be careful using the flashing patterns with people who have epilepsy.

Aims for using the equipment

- To gain a person's attention.
- To provide visual stimulation.
- To teach cause and effect and practise switching skills.
- To learn about colours.

How to use the equipment to stimulate the different senses

Touch

- Not applicable – unless textured switches are used.

Movement

- Encourage people to reach out to the switch to turn on the lights.

Seeing

- Watch the colours moving.
- Look at the different coloured lights.

Hearing

- Not applicable.

Smell

- Not applicable.

Cheaper and everyday alternatives

- Make your own light box using light-emitting diodes (LEDs).
- Cut out spiral shapes in card. Cover the back with different coloured cellophane. Use with an overhead projector or shine a torch through the cellophane.
- Go for a ride in the forest and look at the different lights and shadows created by the trees. Be aware that this can cause some people to have seizures.

 Copyright © Scope (Vic.) Ltd 2008

LADDER LIGHTS

Description

These are vertical columns of different coloured lights, which are sound activated. They can either be used with a sound system or a microphone. As the volume of sound increases, the higher up the ladder the lights travel. When the sound ceases, the lights drop back down to the bottom. There is also a mode where, when the sound ceases, the lights stay at the level they reached. If the sound is louder the next time, the lights will travel even higher up the ladder. There is a sound-sensitivity control, although on some units it does not seem to be sensitive enough to pick up very quiet vocalizations.

PRECAUTION

- Be careful using the flashing lights with people who have epilepsy.

Aims for using the equipment

- To set up a relaxing environment.
- To gain a person's attention.
- To provide visual stimulation.
- To teach cause and effect and practise switching skills.
- To learn about colours.
- To encourage people to vocalize.

How to use the equipment to stimulate the different senses

Touch

- Not applicable – unless textured switches are used to operate the tape-recorder.

Movement

- Encourage people to reach out to the switch to turn on the music.
- Encourage them to point at the different coloured lights.

Seeing

- Watch the colours moving up and down the ladder.

Hearing

- Listen to the sounds of the music and see how it makes the lights travel up the ladder.
- Listen to the volume of vocalizations and how it affects the lights moving up the ladder.

Smell

- Not applicable.

Other ways to use the equipment

- Play quiet music, dim the lights and watch the lights move up and down the ladder in reaction to the music.
- Place the microphone from the ladder lights next to a speaker and use the Soundbeam. When people move in the beam, not only will they create a sound, but they will also see the lights moving.
- Encourage people to vocalize to make the lights move.
- Set up a tape-recorder with power box and switch. Encourage people to use a switch to turn on the music, which will then activate the ladder lights.

Cheaper and everyday alternatives

- Go to the pub and listen to or use the karaoke machine.
- Buy sound-activated equipment.
- Attend a sound and light show.

 Copyright © Scope (Vic.) Ltd 2008

Activities
HEARING

SOUND SYSTEM

Description

When working with sound or choosing CDs, remember that high-frequency sounds can capture a person's attention, while low-frequency sounds are felt through the body. These bass sounds are the ones that are felt most effectively when using a vibroacoustic beanbag or sound box (a unit used with the Soundbeam).

When considering a sound system, look for one with a cassette recorder, radio, multifunction CD player (up to three CDs) and a microphone input so that you can make recordings. It is also useful to buy a system with detachable speakers.

PRECAUTION

- Ensure that all wiring is professionally installed.

Aims for using the equipment

- To provide music to create a relaxing environment.
- To provide music to create a stimulating environment.
- To provide auditory stimulation and show a person's reaction to sound – use everyday sounds, different types of music, people's voices.
- To experiment with sound (e.g. loud/soft, different rhythms).
- To experiment with hearing, listening and making sounds.
- To practise switching skills and teach cause and effect by using the cassette recorder with a switch, through a power box.
- To use sound with the vibroacoustic beanbag/pillow so that people can 'feel' the sounds.

How to use the equipment to stimulate the different senses

Touch

- Not applicable – unless using with a vibroacoustic beanbag.

Movement

- Encourage people to reach out to use the switch to turn the music on.
- Encourage rhythmic movements.

Seeing

- Not applicable.

Copyright © Scope (Vic.) Ltd 2008

Hearing

- Listen to the different types of music – do people have a preference?

Smell

- Not applicable.

Other ways to use the equipment

- Make up tapes with everyday sounds. Use them in a sound lotto game.
- Record people's voices – do people react to the voices of the people they know well (e.g. parents, other family members, other support people)? Do people recognize their own voice and each other's voices?
- Make up a collection of different types of music – for example, rock, classical, country, folk, pop – and collect music from different countries.
- Tape the CDs to use in a cassette player. Use the cassette player with a power box and switch so that people can turn the music on. If a CD is used with the timer on the power box, every time the CD stops and is turned back on, it will reset back to the start of the CD. An electrician can wire up the player to enable the switch to activate the mute or pause button so that the CD doesn't go back to the beginning of the song.

Copyright © Scope (Vic.) Ltd 2008

THE SOUNDBEAM

Description

The Soundbeam is a piece of equipment with an ultrasonic sensor that is attached to a keyboard or sound module. It creates a virtual keyboard or musical instrument in space that can be 'played' through people's movements. As people move through this invisible beam, it triggers the notes or sounds of the keyboard or sound module. This means that people can create interesting sounds even with the smallest movements (see Figure 2.3 p.32).

The Soundbeam can also be accessed through switches, which can trigger individual notes, chords or different sounds.

A vibroacoustic beanbag and sound box can also be purchased to use with the Soundbeam. When people sit in these, they can feel the vibrations created by others moving within the Soundbeam (see Figures 2.5 and 2.6 p.34).

PRECAUTIONS

- Take care when directing the sensor from the Soundbeam so that the beam is not accidentally activated. The aim is for the Soundbeam to be activated by people, not by movement of a table, wall or floor.

- Keep the volume control close at hand and keep the volume down/off when making adjustments. Don't confuse people who will hear sounds being made as the beam is moved while making adjustments, even though they are not moving themselves.

Aims for using the equipment
- To provide auditory stimulation.
- To provide tactile stimulation (from the vibroacoustic beanbag/sound box).
- To provide visual stimulation (when using a shadow screen).
- To encourage people to move.
- To create soundscapes.
- To create performances.
- To teach cause and effect.
- To provide an opportunity to express likes and dislikes in terms of sounds and rhythms.
- To provide an opportunity to make choices.

How to use the equipment to stimulate the different senses
Touch

- Set up the Soundbeam with a sound box or vibroacoustic beanbag.

Movement

- Move in different ways in the Soundbeam. Use different parts of the body to activate the Soundbeam.

Seeing

- Set up the Soundbeam with a projection screen and spotlight. Stand between the light and the projection screen and move within the Soundbeam. People on the other side of the screen will be able to see the shadows of the person working in the Soundbeam (see Figure 2.9 p.35).

Hearing

- Listen to the different sounds created with the Soundbeam.

Smell

- Not applicable.

Other ways to use the equipment

- Drape a fibre-optic spray over a frame and angle the Soundbeam onto it. Encourage people to reach out to the spray. As they reach out, they will activate the Soundbeam.
- Place the microphone from the ladder lights to the speakers attached to the Soundbeam. The lights will activate as people move in the beam and produce different sounds.
- Use the sound effects from the sound module to build up sensory stories. A list of the different sound effects can be found in the Soundbeam manual – for example, a ghost story may use the following sounds: heartbeat, scream, laugh, telephone, door slam and scratch. The Soundbeam can be used with the 'haunted house' set-up and switches can be used to trigger the different sound effects.
- Create a relaxing environment using soothing sounds – for example, 'No. 16 Outer Isle' set-up and relaxing essential oils such as lavender.
- Create a stimulating environment using 'No. 23 Africa' or 'No. 5 percussion' set-ups with uplifting oils (e.g. geranium or peppermint). Remember to consult with an aromatherapist before using essential oils.
- Some people may find it difficult to understand that they need to move in the beam to create a sound, because there is nothing for them to see. Encourage movement by holding out objects for people to reach for (e.g. hoops, balls and scarves).
- Encourage people to move objects in the beam behind the shadow screen for other people to look at. Use co-active assistance if necessary. Create the shadow screen by putting a lamp behind a projection screen made of Lycra®, with the people watching the show sitting on the other side of the screen.
- Make up a large Lycra® bag that people can stand in, or use a white sheet. Encourage people to push out against the bag or sheet while standing in the Soundbeam. People can then pretend to be ghosts in a ghost story (Helen Dilkes).
- Visit the Soundbeam website, www.soundbeam.co.uk, for more information and ideas.

Cheaper and everyday alternatives

- Play some music and have a dance.

- Go to a concert. Remember to think about concerts in the park, jazz at the zoo, etc.

- Attend local festivals, because there will often be bands playing.

- Go and listen to a multicultural choir.

- Listen to a pub band.

- Make shadow puppets and move them behind a projection screen (or large piece of white Lycra®/white curtain).

- Instead of using a sound box, make your own resonance board, so that you can walk on, tap on or drop objects on the board and people can feel the vibrations through the wood.

 Copyright © Scope (Vic.) Ltd 2008

MUSICAL WALLS/FLOORS

Description

Musical walls usually contain a midi box and keyboard. The keyboard can be programmed to play a range of different musical instruments and there are a number of options within that. When a shape or panel is pressed, the wall can play single notes, chords, a sequence of notes, a percussion instrument or sound effects.

There are basically two versions. One has coloured shapes that have to be pressed to get a note or sequence of notes. The other has tactile panels that need to be pressed to get the sound. The tactile version is a more versatile piece of equipment because the sound can be turned off and the wall used purely for its tactile properties. This is also useful because some people may be over-stimulated trying to cope with sound and touch. Figure 5.16 shows a portable tactile musical wall.

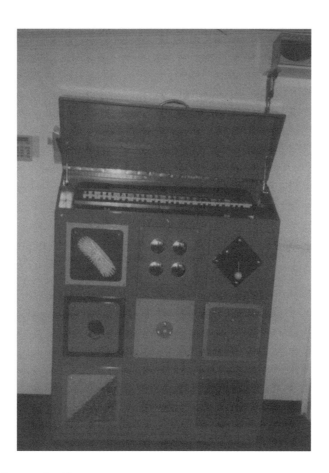

Figure 5.16: A portable tactile musical wall

The musical walls can be used with switches for those who cannot operate the panels directly. Mat switches are particularly useful for those who use gross motor skills to operate the switches. For example, they can roll on the mat switches to operate the musical wall. Tactile covers can be made for mat switches so that people feel different textures when they roll on the mats.

Copyright © Scope (Vic.) Ltd 2008

Some musical walls are also sound light walls, which are sound activated. This means that, when someone vocalizes or music is played, the colours within the wall change, or change in intensity.

A variation on musical walls is musical floors. These can either have tactile cushions that can be leant on, crawled over or sat on to operate the sounds, or they can be linked up to coloured lights. These sound/light walls can either be operated directly, by standing on the floor panels, or through switches.

PRECAUTIONS

- Experiment with the different options and familiarize yourself with the equipment before using it with other people.

- Remember to turn the keyboard on if sound is required from the musical wall.

Aims for using the equipment

- To provide auditory stimulation.
- To find out which sounds people prefer.
- To provide tactile stimulation – feeling the textures of the different tactile panels or tactile switch mat covers.
- To provide visual stimulation – looking at the coloured shapes or textures on the walls.
- To teach cause and effect – when I press a panel/switch, I get a sound.
- To provide an opportunity to make choices – which sound to use/which tactile panel/mat to use.
- To teach shape/colour recognition.

How to use the equipment to stimulate the different senses

Touch

- Make up different tactile mat covers for the mat switches.
- Make up tactile covers for button switches.
- Feel the different textures on the tactile musical wall.

Movement

- Encourage people to reach out to use the switches or operate the panels.
- Use mat switches and encourage people to roll to get the sound from the musical wall.

Copyright © Scope (Vic.) Ltd 2008

Seeing

- Look at the different coloured shapes or textures on the panels.

Hearing

- Listen to the sounds made by operating the different panels or switches.

Smell

- Not applicable.

Cheaper and everyday alternatives

- Buy a keyboard and play/listen to someone playing it.
- Attend a concert.
- Buy CDs of different types of music – for example, piano music, instrumental music, rock and roll, pop, country, jazz, music from different countries.
- Provide auditory stimulation by using wind chimes, sound makers and BIGMacks™.

WIND CHIMES

Description

Wind chimes are objects that are strung together, making a sound when moved by wind. There are a number of different wind chimes that can be bought or made and provide different types of sounds – for example, wooden chimes, metal chimes, small bells.

PRECAUTIONS

- Take care not to hang wind chimes where people can knock their heads on them or get caught up in them.

Aims for using the equipment

- To provide auditory stimulation.
- To provide tactile stimulation – feeling the textures of the different wind chimes.
- To provide visual stimulation – looking at the wind chimes.
- To teach cause and effect (e.g. when I pull this rope, the chimes will make a sound).
- To create a relaxing environment (a fan blowing on small chimes).
- To encourage the people to attend (some people require an auditory cue in order to look at objects).

How to use the equipment to stimulate the different senses

Touch

- Make up different types of wind chime – for example, bamboo, metal pipe, old spoons, kitchen utensils (see Figure 2.9 p.35).
- Feel the wind from a fan directed at the wind chimes.

Movement

- Encourage people to reach out to use the switch on the fan to move the wind chimes.
- Encourage people to reach out to make the wind chimes move.

Seeing

- Use holographic paper or glittery paper on the wind chimes. Direct a spotlight onto the chimes.

Hearing

- Listen to the sounds made by different wind chimes.

Smell

- Not applicable.

 Copyright © Scope (Vic.) Ltd 2008

Other ways to use the equipment

- Wind chimes can be operated manually if they are mounted low enough for people to reach. Wind chimes made from metal pipes are good for this because they are sturdy and can take rough handling. If the chimes are too delicate to handle directly, a rope can be attached to them and pulled to move them. The rope can be made easier to grasp by adding different handles – for example, a spade handle or ball.

- Direct a fan onto the wind chimes so that people can use a switch to operate the fan, which then blows onto the wind chimes to set them moving.

- Direct a spotlight onto the wind chimes to highlight them.

- Use holographic wrapping paper or other glittery paper on the wind chimes. If a spotlight is directed onto them, the light will be reflected by the paper, giving further visual stimulation.

- Make up metal-pipe wind chimes to 'represent' people. Cut lengths of pipe according to the length of people's limbs – for example, shoulder to elbow, elbow to wrist, and hip to knee. These will need to be made in a workshop using goggles and special equipment to cut the metal. Ensure that people are trained in using the equipment and observe correct and safe work practices when using tools. If there is no access to a workshop, then take people's measurements to a workshop and ask them to cut the lengths for you.

- Have a ceiling grid made up and hang wind chimes and other instruments from it.

- Suspend wind chimes on an instrument frame.

Copyright © Scope (Vic.) Ltd 2008

SOUND MAKERS

Description

These are small pieces of equipment powered by either mains electricity or batteries. They have a small selection of sounds, which can be chosen by pressing the corresponding button. The buttons are usually tiny so would be difficult for many people to operate. The sounds are often forest sounds, streams, a summer's night and sometimes a heartbeat and white noise. Some of the sound makers are attached to aromatherapy diffusers so that scented beads can be heated up or oils released from a pad as well as sounds.

Aims for using the equipment

- To provide auditory stimulation and show a person's reaction to the different sounds
- To provide sounds to create a relaxing environment.

How to use the equipment to stimulate the different senses

Touch

- Not applicable.

Movement

- Not applicable.

Seeing

- Not applicable.

Hearing

- Listen to the different types of sound – do people have a preference?

Smell

- Observe people's responses to the different smells.

 Copyright © Scope (Vic.) Ltd 2008

BIGMack

Description

These look like big round switches. They can be used as switches with switch leads. However, they are also single message devices. Record your own sounds by holding down the switch and the record button at the same time. They are useful to assess whether or not people respond to everyday sounds – for example, the telephone, microwave bell – because the sounds can be presented in isolation, without other distracting noises in the same environment. If there is too much going on, it is difficult to assess exactly what the person is responding to.

Aims for using the equipment

- To provide auditory stimulation.
- To provide tactile stimulation if different textures are attached to the BIGMack™.
- To teach cause and effect.
- To match pictures/photographs and textures to sounds.
- To provide an opportunity to make choices – which sounds to use.

How to use the equipment to stimulate the different senses

Touch

- Add textures to the top of the BIGMack™ and feel them when operating the switch. Feel the textures or look at pictures secured on the BIGMack™. Also use glittery paper/holographic paper on the switches. Put white paper on the switch and use under UV light. Use clear Perspex™ caps that clip over the top of the switch to keep paper and pictures in place. Velcro® could also be added to the clear caps so that different textures could be attached to these rather than to the switches themselves.

Movement

- Encourage people to reach out and operate the BIGMack™.

Seeing

- Look at pictures secured on the BIGMack™. Use clear Perspex™ caps that clip over the top of the switch to keep paper and pictures in place. Also use glittery paper/holographic paper on the switches. Put white paper on the switch and use under UV. Velcro® could also be added to the clear caps so that different textures could be attached to these rather then the switches themselves.

Hearing

- Listen to the sounds from the BIGMack™.

Smell

- Not applicable.

Copyright © Scope (Vic.) Ltd 2008

Other ways to use the equipment

- Use it to record individual people's vocalizations. When played back, it is interesting to see how people respond to their own sounds.

- Use to record repetitive phrases for a story (e.g. *Three Little Pigs, Not by the Hair of My Chinny Chin Chin.*

- Collect objects to go with the sounds – for example, a teaspoon in a teacup – and play a game matching the sounds to the objects.

- Take the BIGMacks™ to the beach and record different sounds – for example, the sound of waves, seagulls squawking – and use in a sensory story.

- Place different textures on the BIGMacks™ so that when people operate the switch they also get to feel something. Think about matching the texture to the sound (e.g. feather to bird sound, blue cellophane to waterfall/stream, lamb's wool to the sound of a lamb, suede to the sound of a cow).

- Place pictures of the sounds on the BIGMacks™ so that people can choose the sound they want from the picture. Play picture/sound-matching games.

Cheaper and everyday alternatives

- Try recording different voices and sounds onto a tape or CD. Play it back and see if people recognise their voices. To make the activity more interactive, plug the tape or CD player into a Powerbox and turn on using a switch.

 Copyright © Scope (Vic.) Ltd 2008

Activities
SMELL

AROMA DIFFUSERS

Description

These are pieces of equipment using a heat source to warm up oils so that their aroma is released. It is recommended that an electric/battery-operated aromatherapy diffuser is used rather than one that heats oils with a candle. There is always the risk that a candle can be knocked over and start a fire.

There are a number of different types of aromatherapy diffuser – one that just heats a ceramic dish, another that also incorporates a fan to spread the smells around the room, and one that forms a plug that is plugged into a mains socket. There are also combination units which incorporate aromatherapy diffusers with different relaxing sounds, such as a babbling brook or forest sounds.

The companies that supply equipment for multisensory rooms also supply the aromatherapy diffusers. However, these are also readily available from large department stores.

Variations on the aromatherapy diffuser are smell tubes/boxes. These either use aromatherapy oils or vials of smells. The vials can contain a variety of everyday smells, pleasant and unpleasant, such as cut grass or manure. However, remember where possible to try to experience the natural smells.

PRECAUTIONS

- If using eucalyptus plugs, be aware that the strong smell could be overwhelming for some people.

- If using an aroma diffuser with a ceramic dish, remember to clean it regularly. The oils leave a sticky residue when they heat up.

- If using an aroma diffuser with a pad that absorbs oils, use different pads for different oils; otherwise, the mix of smells could be unpleasant.

- Remember to disconnect the unit from the power supply before changing the cartridge or pad.

- Don't use more than two or three smells in a session because people can become overwhelmed or unable to distinguish the different smells any more.

- Only use a few drops of oil because the aromas can be overpowering. Remember that some people may be sensitive to different smells that might make them feel ill. Remember to observe people carefully and note their reactions to the different oils.

- Remember to consult with an aromatherapist on the types of oils and how to use them with people.

Copyright © Scope (Vic.) Ltd 2008

Aims for using the equipment

- Use it with other equipment (e.g. quiet music to set up an environment for relaxation).
- Offer the opportunity to make choices, e.g. which scent to use.
- Use other oils (e.g. citrus oil) to create a stimulating environment.
- Use it to create particular environments (e.g. manure smell for a farmyard).
- Use it to stimulate the sense of smell.

How to use the equipment to stimulate the different senses

Touch

- Feel the vibrations from the aromatherapy diffusers that also incorporate a fan.

Movement

- Encourage people to move the smell tubes to waft the smells around the room and in front of the nose.

Seeing

- Not applicable.

Hearing

- Listen to the hum from the powered aroma diffusers. Are people distracted by the noise?

Smell

- Smell the different scents.

Other ways to use the equipment

- Use different smells in different parts of the house, school or centre to indicate the activity that takes place in different rooms (e.g. pine for the toilet, lemon for the kitchen, lavender for the lounge room).
- Use different smells to indicate different days of the week (e.g. an uplifting oil for weekdays and a relaxing oil for the weekends).

Copyright © Scope (Vic.) Ltd 2008

Cheaper and everyday alternatives

- Go for a walk in the garden after the grass has been cut.
- Visit a farm.
- Visit a herb garden.
- Grow your own herbs.
- Make pot pourri and lavender bags.
- Visit a garden and smell the flowers.
- Buy a bread maker and make your own bread – smell the bread cooking.
- Make your own carpet freshener (bicarbonate of soda with drops of essential oils).
- Use lemon-scented washing-up liquid and wash the dishes.
- Buy scented bubble bath to use in the bath.
- Use scented shower gel in the shower.
- Make your own lemon juice and smell the lemons.
- Make up 'smell' bottles. Use pop-top drink bottles with tops that pop up and click down to close. Put small stones/glass beads in the bottom to almost fill the bottle. Put essential oils on balls of cotton wool and put these at the top of the bottle. Pull the pop-top up to experience the smell in the bottle. Push the top down to keep the smell inside the bottle.
- Buy the plugs with the vapour pads/liquid used to help breathing when you have a cold.
- Buy the plugs for wall sockets which release aromatherapy oils or other house freshener scents.

 Copyright © Scope (Vic.) Ltd 2008

6

Multisensory Stories and Themes

Introduction

This last chapter of the book outlines ideas for sensory themes and sensory stories. I have been using the multisensory rooms as multisensory theatres. People appear to enjoy the structure of the story and adding in the names of the people in the group can customize it. Solar effects wheels can also be made with photos of the participants, which is always motivating.

Different ideas for stories are outlined here and the sensory components of the story are highlighted. The outline is set out in the form of bullet list: the equipment required is listed, together with ideas for the different senses. Use this as a guide to make your own sensory stories. Remember to assess people with single stimuli to ensure that they can cope with multisensory work.

For other ideas on multisensory themes and stories, think about making up stories based on activities people do – for example, a trip to the beach/park – and important events in their lives. Also think about the seasons, special events, bible stories, fairy stories, Aesop's fables, Greek mythology, Aboriginal dreamtime stories, African stories and other cultural tales. If you do not know any stories, think about using the internet. Type in a topic such as Aesop's fables (remember the story about the tortoise and the hare?) and you will be able to find information about the different stories. When looking for multisensory stories, think about the sensory properties of the story. Are there enough different sensory objects in the story for use as a multisensory theme or story? Also consider the different senses – how can they be incorporated into the story? Use art and craft sessions to make objects for multisensory themes. When visiting places in the local community, look out for items that can be used in a multisensory theme.

Included within this chapter are two scripts that show how a particular story can be represented.

AN ADVENTURE ON THE HIGH SEAS

The day could start as a fun day out going on a boat to an outlying island for a picnic. People spend the day exploring the beach and enjoying the picnic. On the way back, the sky turns dark and the boat is caught in a storm. The boat battles through the waves but eventually comes out of the storm and everybody arrives home safely.

Equipment required

- Vibrating mat/cushion
- Leaf chair
- Vibroacoustic beanbag/bed
- Hammock
- Plant sprays
- Different types of marine animals and beach material
- Fish/bird kites
- Chocolate or chocolate mouse

- Projector
- Kites
- Green cellophane, blue material and white tulle
- Sound system
- Salt
- CDs/cassette tapes of bird and whale songs, sounds of the ocean

How to use the story/theme to stimulate the different senses

Touch

- Use plant sprays to spray mists of water to represent the sea spray.
- Feel pieces of seaweed or green cellophane to represent seaweed. Feel different types of shells, warm sand, bowls of water. Feel different textured marine animals – for example, octopus, whale, shark, fish. Use items to represent sea life – for example, koosh ball for sea anemones.

Movement

- Place a person on a vibrating mat or cushion. Vary the settings to represent sailing on calm seas and during a storm.
- Use the leaf chair, vibroacoustic beanbag/bed or hammock to represent being on a boat.

Seeing

- Project an image of whales and seagulls onto the wall. Hang up fish and bird kites.
- Drape blue material and white tulle around the boat (vibrating mat) to represent waves.

Hearing

- Play sounds of birds and whale songs.
- Play ocean sounds.

Copyright © Scope (Vic.) Ltd 2008

Smell

- Smell seaweed, starfish (dried), shells.

Taste

- Chocolate to represent rations, salt for the sea spray.

THE FOREST

Take a walk in the garden/forest/bush to collect leaves.

Equipment required

- Different type of forest material, e.g. leaves, branches, needles, moss
- Camouflage nets
- Bottles
- Leaf chair
- Hammock
- Ceiling grid
- Bowls
- Scented leaves and wood
- Art materials
- Solar projector
- BIGMack™
- Sound makers
- Pine-scented car fresheners
- Picnic food
- Sandalwood/cedarwood oil
- Cotton wool balls

How to use the story/theme to stimulate the different senses

Touch

- Feel different branches, leaves and moss.
- Put some dried leaves in a bowl to feel and scrunch.
- Feel camouflage nets.

Movement

- Move through a bottle forest. Hang the bottles close together so that people have to push their way through.
- Sit in a leaf chair or hammock to represent swinging off the branches, swinging on vines.

Seeing

- Make up a mobile using leaves.
- Thread leaves together and hang off a ceiling grid or netting.
- Make up the 'bottle' forest by decorating empty drinks bottles with glittery contact or bright paint/stickers and suspend from the ceiling.
- Make up a tree wheel to use with the solar projector using real leaves, clip art, photos or drawings of trees.

Hearing

- Use a BIGMack™ to record sounds of the birds, wind in the trees, streams, waterfalls, leaves rustling, rain.
- Use the sound makers that often have forest sounds, streams, waterfalls.

    Copyright © Scope (Vic.) Ltd 2008

Smell

- Hang up pine-scented car fresheners.
- Gather together fresh pine needles.
- Collect other scented leaves and wood – for example, eucalyptus, pine, wet leaves.

Taste

- Have a picnic.

GO FOR A RIDE ON A MOTORBIKE THROUGH THE FOREST

Equipment required

- Massage belt
- Vibriting mats
- Vibroacoustic beanbags
- Pine cones, dried leaves
- Hammock
- Hurricane tube
- Fragrances/essential oils

- Pine-scented car freshener
- Lycra® screen
- Green and brown streamers
- Sound system
- Art materials
- Picnic food

How to use the story/theme to stimulate the different senses

Touch

- Encourage people to hold vibrating equipment – for example, a massage belt to represent the motorbike handlebars.
- Sit/lie on vibrating mats, vibroacoustic beanbags.
- Find pine cones to feel.
- Fill a bowl with dried leaves and feel them.

Movement

- Lie in a hammock to represent moving on the motorbike.

Seeing

- Turn on the hurricane tube and watch the shadows on the ceiling (shadows through the trees).
- Look at shadows behind a Lycra® screen.
- Sit inside a beach tent and hang green and brown streamers from the roof. Put the fan on them and watch them moving.
- Hang large bird and butterfly mobiles.

Hearing

- Listen to the sound of the wind or bird songs – for example, *Dinner in the Daintree* tape or CD.

     Copyright © Scope (Vic.) Ltd 2008

Smell

- Make flowers from people's hand prints (use material or paper). Make up a centre for the flower with cotton wool and put fragrances or essential oil on the wool.
- Smell a pine-scented car freshener.

Taste

- At the end of the ride, stop for a picnic.

THE JOURNEY

The following is a script that could be modified and used with the motorbike ride. The written script is recorded and then paused as people are given the opportunity to experience the sensory elements of the story.

Equipment required

- Vibrating massage
- Projector wheel
- Drums
- Wave drum
- Water spray
- Aroma diffuser
- Pine car fresheners
- Bag of pine needles
- Rubber frog/furry animal
- Coloured feathers
- Fan with power box and switch

- Music tapes
- White lace
- Sticks
- Rain stick
- Fresh flowers
- Incense sticks
- Pine cones, tree bark
- Bowl of dried leaves
- Dinner in the Daintree tape
- Blue silky material on table
- Lavender in pot

(If people are able to, get them to blow the feathers. Alternatively, more able people can wave the material around to make the birds 'fly').

The feathers on the blue silk are an idea I found in Flo Longhorn's *Sensory Drama for Very Special People* (2001).

> We're going on a journey, where shall we go?
> Let's get on the bus and head for the...forest.
> We'll put on our favourite music to help us on the journey.
>
> PAUSE:
> *[Feel vibrating objects to represent vibrations for the bus. Use solar projector to project images of people's faces onto the wall or project pictures of the forest.]*
>
> Oh no, there's a storm coming. Can you see the clouds?
>
> PAUSE:
> *[Wave white lace over people for clouds. Bang drums – thunder, sticks – lightning cracks, wave drum and rain sticks for rain. Spray water for rain. Start off quietly then crescendo for a storm.]*
>
> Phew, that's lucky, it was only a quick storm, now we can get out of the bus.
> The rain has really brought out the smell of the trees. Can you smell them?
>
> PAUSE:
> *Offer people the opportunity to smell the following: fresh flowers; aroma diffuser with forest smells; incense sticks or pine car fresheners.*

Copyright © Scope (Vic.) Ltd 2008

Look over there, what's that? Oh it's a pine cone. Can you feel how rough it is? What else is rough? Oh yes, the tree bark and even the pine needles are spiky and rough. These leaves don't feel rough but they make a lovely crunchy sound. What's that hiding under the leaves?

PAUSE:

Offer people the opportunity to feel: pine cones; bag of pine needles; tree bark; dried leaves and a rubber frog/furry animal – hidden in bowl of leaves.

Shh, be quiet, can you hear the birds? Look how colourful they are; see, they're flying away.

PAUSE:

Change tape/CD to Dinner in the Daintree *tape. Offer people the opportunity to look at coloured feathers and blue silky material on the table. Use the fan with a power box and switch to blow off feathers. Put the original tape back in.*

It's time to go home; let's take a different route back to the bus. How about walking through that lavender patch? Doesn't it smell wonderful and feel so soft?

PAUSE:

Offer people the opportunity to smell and feel lavender in the pot.

Here we are, back at the bus. Let's put the music back on and go back home. It's been a great day.

[Keep tape going so that people can listen to the music ending the journey. Offer people the opportunity to feel the vibrating objects and listen to the music.]

SET UP A SENSORY CORNER WITH A FISH THEME

Use a themed corner to carry out the story of the rainbow fish.

Equipment required

- Streamers
- Fish mobiles and kites
- Fan
- Containers of gravel and sand
- Bowls of water

- Art materials
- Cuttlefish bone
- Sound system
- Seaweed, starfish and shells
- Rice and seaweed savouries

How to use the story/theme to stimulate the different senses

Touch

- Hang up streamers and fish mobiles. Direct a fan onto them. Position people near enough to feel the streamers and material from the fish.
- Position people near enough to feel the breeze.
- Fill different containers with gravel and sand so that people can feel the different textures with their hands and feet.
- Fill bowls of water for people to feel with their hands and feet.
- Make up animals from different textures – for example, seahorse, octopus.
- Find a cuttlefish bone to feel.
- Make up a rainbow fish with different types of silver and holographic paper to feel.

Movement

- Lie in a hammock or on a vibroacoustic beanbag/mat to represent moving in the sea.

Seeing

- Attach bright fish kites in front of the streamers.
- Attach long foil and blue cellophane streamers to the wall/ceiling.
- Put the fan behind the streamers so that the breeze blows through the streamers and moves the fish.
- Play music with the sounds of the sea.
- Listen to the sounds of seagulls.

Copyright © Scope (Vic.) Ltd 2008

Smell/touch

- Offer dried seaweed, dried starfish and shells to feel and smell.
- Collect seaweed to feel and smell.

Taste

- Eat Japanese seaweed. Make rice and seaweed savouries (sushi). Remember to check whether or not people can cope with eating seaweed/rice.

Copyright © Scope (Vic.) Ltd 2008

CREATE A STORY AROUND KING NEPTUNE OR THE LITTLE MERMAID

Equipment required

- Ball pool
- Plaster of Paris
- Crown/treasure chest
- Water
- Plant sprays
- Bubble machines
- White netting

- Projector
- Art materials
- Bird kites
- Sound system
- Soundbeam
- Shells
- Party/banquet food

How to use the story/theme to stimulate the different senses

Touch

- People to sit in the ball pool to represent the water.
- Make plaster of Paris shells.
- Feel a crown, have a treasure chest full of items.
- Feel and explore water. Place items in the water to be found.
- Use plant sprays to simulate water spray from the sea.
- Blow bubbles or use bubble machines so that the bubbles land on people. Use the bubbles to represent sea spray.

Movement

- Sit in a leaf chair or hammock to simulate being rocked in the sea.

Seeing

- Create a frame around the ball pool from which to drape white netting. Project images of fish onto the netting.
- Look at the jewels and items in the crown and treasure chest.
- Make/buy bird kites.

Hearing

- Play music of dolphin songs and waves.
- Have the sound of a storm.
- Use the Soundbeam to create the sound of a storm.
- Have the sound of a choir singing (mermaids' concert).

 Copyright © Scope (Vic.) Ltd 2008

Smell

- Collect shells from the beach to feel and smell.

Taste

- Have a party or banquet; choose food as appropriate.

THE HAUNTED HOUSE

Equipment required

- Threads/string
- Lycra® bag
- Tape-recorder
- Power box
- Mat switches
- Thick card, dowel and art materials
- Projector
- Smoke machine
- Soundbeam
- Stocks
- Musty oils

How to use the story/theme to stimulate the different senses

Touch

- Feel different tactile objects such as furry spiders, bats and cobwebs made from different threads/string.

Movement

- Stand/sit inside a Lycra® bag and push out against the Lycra® to represent ghosts.
- Record sounds of footsteps on a tape cassette and link it to a power box. Encourage people to roll on mat switches or go over them in their wheelchairs to set off the sounds of footsteps.

Seeing

- Watch the shadows created by people moving inside the Lycra® bag.
- Create silhouettes of haunted houses, bats etc. Use thick card to draw out the different shapes and attach to a piece of dowel. Move the shapes behind the projection screen.
- Hire a smoke machine.

Hearing

- Use the ghostly sound set-ups on the Soundbeam.
- Use the sound effects from the keyboard/sound module to create a story. The keyboard/sound module manual will have a list of available sounds – for example, heart beat, scream, laugh, telephone, door slam, scratch.
- Encourage people to stamp feet, tap on sides of wheelchair, use sticks to tap on a table to represent footsteps in the house.

Smell

- Use musty oils – for example, cedarwood.

Taste

- Anything you associate with a haunted house e.g. marshmallows, icy poles or ice cream (cold spooky environment).

 Copyright © Scope (Vic.) Ltd 2008

A NIGHT OUT AT A JAZZ CLUB

Equipment required

- Musical mat and wall
- Mat switches
- Soundbeam
- Differen textured clothes, hat and gloves
- UV lamp

- Sound system
- Jazz music
- Perfumes and aftershave
- Different types of drinks and dips

How to use the story/theme to stimulate the different senses

Touch

- Feel different textured clothes, hat and gloves to wear going out to the club.

Movement

- Encourage people to roll on the different parts of a musical mat. Reach out for the different panels on a musical wall to operate the sounds.
- Roll on mat switches to turn on different types of jazz music.
- Play different types of jazz music by moving through the Soundbeam.

Seeing

- Wear glitter hats to the club.
- Look at white and fluorescent objects under UV light.

Hearing

- Listen to the different sounds from the musical wall.
- Listen to jazz music on CDs.

Smell

- Smell different perfumes and aftershave.

Taste

- Taste different types of drinks and dips.

Copyright © Scope (Vic.) Ltd 2008

KING MIDAS

King Midas was a very rich king, but he could never get enough gold. One day, a strange man arrived in his kingdom and offered the king anything he wanted. The king was excited and asked that everything he touched should turn to gold. The strange man told him that in the morning his wish would be granted.

As soon as the sun rose the next morning, King Midas rushed out of bed and started touching things in his room. He touched a stool and it turned to gold; he then touched a mirror. He also touched the water in the bowl he used for washing. He touched everything in his room, then decided to go down for breakfast. He reached for some fruit, but every piece turned to gold. He reached for his wine, but it turned to gold. The king then decided he wasn't hungry so he went for a walk in his garden instead. On his way out, he touched the wind chimes hanging outside the window. Out in the garden, he found his daughter smelling flowers and exclaiming how wonderful the trees and flowers looked, with all their different colours. The king told her he could make them even better and started touching the trees and flowers, turning them to gold. His daughter was very upset and ran off, but the king was too busy changing everything to gold to notice. He was now with the animals, turning the birds, lambs and dogs to gold. Later in the day, the king saw his daughter crying and went to comfort her. As soon as he touched her, she turned to gold. The king loved his daughter and in that instant he realized that there were more important things than gold.

Equipment required

- Metal crown
- Cardboard, gold paper and art materials
- Lambs wool, fur
- Wood
- Mirror
- Water
- Fruit
- Papier mâché
- Doll/puppet
- Sound system
- Branch sceptre with pine smell
- Different flowers
- Grapes/grape juice

How to use the story/theme to stimulate the different senses

Touch

- Feel the crown – buy a metal one or make one from cardboard covered with gold paper. Lamb's wool for the lamb, fur for the dog, wood for the stool, a mirror.
- Wash hands in water.
- Feel different types of fruit.
- Make up papier mâché fruit.
- Use a doll/puppet to represent the daughter.

Movement

- Encourage people to reach up and ring the wind chimes. Have wind chimes hung at different heights so that people can use arms or legs to operate the wind chimes.

 Copyright © Scope (Vic.) Ltd 2008

Seeing

- Look at different types of gold paper.
- Cover the different objects with gold paper after King Midas has touched them.

Hearing

- Listen to bird songs.
- Listen to the wind chimes.
- Listen to the sound of water being splashed, river sounds.

Smell

- Branch sceptre with pine smell.
- Smell different flowers.

Taste

- Taste grapes/grape juice.
- Taste different types of fruit.

Copyright © Scope (Vic.) Ltd 2008

CLEOPATRA'S BARGE

Queen Cleopatra is surveying her kingdom from her barge. It is a hot and windy day in Egypt. While on the barge, she has a feast and entertainment in the form of music and belly dancing.

Equipment required

- Fabrics
- Hammock
- Bowls of sand and water
- Fan
- Foil
- Spotlight
- Survival blanket
- Incense
- Art materials
- UV lamp
- Projector
- Sound system
- Egiptian music
- Small bells
- Scarf
- Small coins
- Ingredients for Turkish Delight and Baklava

How to use the story/theme to stimulate the different senses

Touch

- Use different fabrics to drape around the hammock – for example, chiffon scarves, lace.
- Bowls of sand and water to feel.
- Direct the wind from the fan onto the fabrics to represent the wind.
- Use sandalwood fans, fans made from feathers.
- Feel purple sails and silver (foil) oars.

Movement

- Sit in the hammock to represent being on the barge. Ensure that people are secure and don't fall out.

Seeing

- Shine a spotlight onto a survival blanket to represent the sun.
- Make up a painting with pyramids and camels. Use fluorescent paint to glow under UV light, make up a wheel with pyramids and camels, or project slides with an Egyptian theme.

Hearing

- Play Egyptian music.
- Find small bells and mount them so that the wind from the fan blows on them or they ring when the hammock moves.
- Wrap a scarf with small coins around people (used for belly dancing).

 Copyright © Scope (Vic.) Ltd 2008

Smell

- Burn some incense in the room before people come in. Leave it on long enough so that the smell lingers. But be very careful using incense and don't leave it unattended.

Taste

- Make Turkish Delight and try Baklava. Check with a speech pathologist first because Baklava has nuts in it.

JONAH AND THE WHALE

Jonah went on a ship to flee from God who had asked him to go to Nineveh to cry out against the wickedness there. God sent a great wind and tempest to break the ship that Jonah was on. The sailors threw their wares overboard to make the ship lighter so that it wouldn't sink. Jonah said that he should be thrown over as well as it was because of him there was a storm. Once he was cast in the sea, it became calm and a whale swallowed him. When inside the whale, Jonah repented and turned back to God, so the whale spat him out onto dry land.

Equipment required

- Different fish and sea creatures
- Art materials, including green cellophane and fluorescent paint
- Water bed/lilo
- Hammock
- Vibroacoustic beanbag/bed

- Effects wheel
- UV lamp

- Sound system
- Seaweed
- Fish and chips

How to use the story/theme to stimulate the different senses

Touch

- Make and buy different fish and sea creatures. Feel the different textures.
- In the art room, feel a real fish and make fish prints.
- Make a tactile whale.
- Feel green cellophane to represent seaweed.

Movement

- Move on the waterbed/lilo, hammock or vibroacoustic beanbag/bed to represent being inside the whale.

Seeing

- Make up an effects wheel and project images of fish, seaweed, etc. or use 'the deep' effects wheel.
- Paint small fish in fluorescent paint and view under UV light.

Hearing

- Play music of whales and dolphins.
- Listen to the sounds of the sea.

 Copyright © Scope (Vic.) Ltd 2008

Smell

- Smell seaweed and fish.

Taste

- Eat fish and chips.

TREASURE ISLAND

One service used the fibre-optic spray as a prop in their story of *Treasure Island*. They made a tape of an abbreviated version of the story and incorporated the following sensory elements into it. The script is included here.

Equipment required

- Bowls of sand
- Parachute
- Shells and starfish
- Captain's chest with contents related to the story
- Treasure chest with contents related to the story
- Leaf chair
- Hammock
- Lilo

- Fibre optics
- Red collophane
- Power box and switch
- Mat switches
- UV paint and lamp
- Projector wheel
- Sound system
- Chocolate coins

How to use the story/theme to stimulate the different senses

Touch

- Feel bowls of sand to represent the beach.
- Wave a parachute overhead to represent the wind in the sails of the ship.
- Put shells and starfish in the sand to provide another texture to feel.
- Feel contents of the captain's chest – for example, a silk shirt, leather boots, jacket with braids and golden buttons, bag of coins, a map on a piece of chamois.
- Feel (and look at) contents of the treasure chest – for example, chocolate coins, tiara, coloured glass stones (used in flower vases), silver coloured cutlery, teapot, etc.

Movement

- Swing in a leaf chair or hammock to represent being on a boat.
- Lay a person on a lilo and move the air in the lilo to move the person to represent being on a boat.

Seeing

- Place fibre optics underneath red cellophane. Connect fibre optics to a power box and switch so that people can turn on the 'fire'. Remember to also use mat switches so that people can roll on and off the mat to light up the 'fire'.
- Paint skull and crossbones flag in UV paint. Observe under UV light.
- Make up a projector wheel with a yellow special effects wheel to represent the moon.

 Copyright © Scope (Vic.) Ltd 2008

Hearing

- Listen to a recording of a sea shanty (song).
- Listen to the sound of the waves.
- Listen to the sound of dolphins, seagulls.

Smell

- Not applicable

Taste

- Eat the chocolate coins.

Treasure Island script

This is the story of Treasure Island as told by young Jim Hawkins after his return from his great adventure, a tale of treachery and terror. It all began a long time ago in England at the Admiral Benbow Inn where Jim Hawkins lived with his parents.

A weather-beaten sailor known as the Captain arrived at the Inn one day with an old sea chest. Every evening, he sat in front of the fire in the parlour drinking rum and singing his favourite song.

[Everyone takes turns to turn on a switch which is connected to the power board and optic fibres to see the fire – which is red cellophane with the fibres under them.]

The Captain sings:

> Fifteen men on a dead man's chest
> Yo-ho-ho and a bottle of rum
> Drink and the devil be done with the rest
> Yo-ho-ho and a bottle of rum…

Every day, he would go down to the beach to look for ships on the sea through his spyglass. He would sit on the cliffs listening to the waves beating on the rocks and feel the sand with his fingers.

[Listen to the waves, and get people to put their hands into the sand and shells and feel them like the Captain. (5 minutes)]

One day, the old Captain died. It was then that an old blind beggar came looking for him. Jim Hawkins was afraid of Pew the beggar and sneaked upstairs to look in the Captain's sea chest. Jim Hawkins found lots of interesting things. Let's feel them and guess what they are.

Copyright © Scope (Vic.) Ltd 2008

[Pass the items in the wooden chest around one item at a time so that people can feel the different textures – for example:

- a soft silk shirt
- leather boots
- a jacket with braids and golden buttons
- a bag of coins
- a map on a piece of chamois.

(10 minutes)]

Did you find a soft shirt? Did you feel the gold braid on the Captain's jacket? Did you find the gold coins?

Jim was very excited about finding the gold coins too, but suddenly there was a banging on the door [banging] and pirates came running in wanting to have the Captain's sea chest [noise and shouting – bring us the sea chest and the treasure].

Jim Hawkins ran away holding onto the map that he had found in the bottom of the chest. Jim Hawkins met up with his friends and they all boarded a ship to sail to Treasure Island to find the buried treasure that was drawn on the Captain's map.

The ship had sails that billowed in the wind, and Jim Hawkins and his friends stayed on the ship for a long time listening to the wind and waves and feeling the sails moving. Can you imagine being on the ship too?

[Listen to the waves and the wind. Move the parachute over people to give the feeling of the billowing sails. (3–4 minutes)]

> Fifteen men on a dead man's chest
> Yo-ho-ho and a bottle of rum
> Drink and the devil be done with the rest
> Yo-ho-ho and a bottle of rum…

The pirates had caught up with Jim Hawkins and his friends – they could see the pirates' flag flapping from the mast of their ship – it looked scary and Jim Hawkins and his friends shook with fear and jumped overboard and swam to Treasure Island.

[Turn on the UV light, highlighting the skull and crossbones flag that is hung underneath. At the same time, dim the main light. Try and encourage people to look at the flag. (1 minute)]

Copyright © Scope (Vic.) Ltd 2008

Jim Hawkins and his friends had many adventures as they followed the clues on the map in searching for the Captain's treasure chest on Treasure Island. The whole time that they were on Treasure Island, the pirates chased them in the race to find the treasure first. Jim Hawkins and his friends had to hide in the woods on the island after having a fight with the pirates. They hid among the trees for a long time until the stars finally came out and the large golden moon rose so that they could find their way back to the beach.

[Dim the lights. Turn on the projector with the yellow special effects wheel to portray the moonlight.]

As Jim Hawkins and his friends hunted around on the beach among some trees, they found a cave hidden in the greenery – it was almost covered in vines that had grown there for a long time. Jim Hawkins and his friends went into the cave and began digging in the sand. Soon they hit something hard hidden under the sand [clinking sound]. They uncovered an old chest that had lain under the sand for many years. As Jim Hawkins and his friends dragged the old chest out, they were very excited and began cheering [hurrah]. WAS this what they had been searching for all this time? They slowly opened the chest [creak] WHAT DO YOU THINK THEY FOUND...?

[Take the small chest around to each person so that they can look inside and take out a piece of the treasure. After a few minutes of looking and feeling the treasure, get people to put the treasure back in the chest.]

THE END

Treasure Island idea courtesy of Brigitte Mcdonald
from Interact Learning Centre, Victoria.

CENTRE PIECE FOR BEACH THEME/'A DAY AT THE BEACH' STORY

Equipment required

- Sand, shells, seaweed, starfish
- Cellophane, silver paper and art materials
- Fan
- Wheat bags
- Sun-tan lotion and aloe vera gel
- Hammock
- Leaf chair
- Vibrating mat
- Spotlight
- Soundbeam
- Fruit and vegetables
- Juice extractor

- Plastic fish
- Bubble tube
- Effect wheel
- Projector
- Survival blanket
- White umbrella
- Fish prints, mobiles and kites
- Sound system
- Aromatherapy diffuser
- Coconut essence and sun lotion
- Fish and chips
- Ice-cream

How to use the story/theme to stimulate the different senses

Touch

- Make tactile sea creatures, collect sand, shells, seaweed. Feel dried starfish.
- Feel the wind from a fan and heat from a wheat bag.
- Make 'seaweed' with strips of cellophane.
- Warm up some of the sand and feel the difference between warm and cold sand.
- Feel hot wheat packs.
- Hide shells in the sand. Add water to the sand and feel the difference.
- Feel and smell sun-tan lotion and aloe vera gel (for sunburn).

Movement

- Lie in a hammock or leaf chair, or sit on a vibrating mat (getting a massage on the beach).
- Set up objects that encourage people to want to reach out and move their arms – for example, hang up silver paper and blue cellophane. Direct a spotlight onto the silver paper to make it visually attractive, or make a 'beach mobile' by gluing sand onto card.
- Use swimming movements within the Soundbeam to create the sounds of waves crashing on the beach, or bird sounds.

 Copyright © Scope (Vic.) Ltd 2008

Centre piece for beach theme/ 'A day at the beach' story (see story outline in Appendix 8) CONTINUED

Seeing

- Put plastic fish in the bubble tube and watch them moving in the bubbles.
- Make up an effects wheel of a surfer and project it onto blue cloth.
- Recreate the sun – project light onto a survival blanket (glare of sun) or project yellow light.
- Project beach images onto a white umbrella (sunshade).
- Decorate room with fish prints, fish mobiles and kites.
- Project images onto plain kites.

Hearing

- Crumple the cellophane seaweed, listen to the sound of waves, dolphins, wind from a fan, seagulls, beach songs – for example, by the Beachboys.
- Hug the bubble tube and rest your ear against the tube to listen to the gurgling of the sea.
- Use the Soundbeam to create a sound atmosphere – for example, wave sounds, birdsong.
- Make a wind chime from shells; direct the fan onto the shells to set them moving.

Smell

- Use an aromatherapy diffuser with beach smells – e.g coconut. Smell coconut essence, coconut sun lotion, seaweed, sun-tan lotion and aloe vera gel.

Taste

- Go out for fish and chips and ice-cream.
- Make coconut ice (be aware that some people have difficulties eating coconut). Use a juice extractor with a switch to make up different types of fruit and vegetable juice – e.g. water melon, banana, pineapple, carrots.

Copyright © Scope (Vic.) Ltd 2008

A CHRISTMAS CAROL

Ebenezer Scrooge is a miser, whose only interest is in hoarding money. He detests Christmas and everyone being happy around him. One Christmas Eve, he is visited by three ghosts of Christmas – past, present and future – who make him see how mean he has been. In the morning Scrooge reforms, sending gifts and spending time with his family.

Children may prefer the story of the Grinch who stole Christmas.

Equipment required

- Christmas decorations
- Net bags
- Paper hats
- Felt bags
- Christmas stockings
- Card, gold paper and art materials
- Costume material
- Hurricane tube
- Sound system

- Small bells
- Fan
- Crackers
- Cinnamon sticks
- Sandpaper
- Christmas puddings, mince pies, shortbread
- Chocolate gold chains

How to use the story/theme to stimulate the different senses

Touch

- Feel different Christmas decorations. Put small decorations inside a net bag – for example, laundry bag or orange bag.
- Feel paper hats.
- Feel felt bags and other textures on Christmas stockings.
- Feel large gold coins made from card and gold paper.
- Put marbles in a bag and encourage people to feel the money bag.
- Feel the material of costumes for the ghosts.

Movement

- Walk or push wheelchairs around the room to visit friends and family, distributing gifts.

Seeing

- Watch the tinsel balls moving in the hurricane tube.

Hearing

- Listen to Christmas carols.
- Hang up small bells and encourage people to operate the switch to the fan to make the bells chime.
- Pull crackers and listen to the bang.

 Copyright © Scope (Vic.) Ltd 2008

Smell

- Make up a cinnamon star mobile by scratching cinnamon sticks onto sandpaper and then cutting out the shapes.

Taste

- Make and eat Christmas pudding, mince pies, shortbread.
- Eat chocolate gold coins.

Copyright © Scope (Vic.) Ltd 2008

BONFIRE NIGHT

Equipment required

- Fabric of warm clothes
- Materials for making a Guy Fawkes
- Sticks and dried leaves
- Fibre-optic spray
- Red, orange and yellow cellophane
- Blue acetate
- Overhead projector

- Sound system
- Sparklers
- Clothes with smell of smoke from a wood fire
- Hot chocolate
- Toffee apples

How to use the story/theme to stimulate the different senses

Touch

- Feel the fabric of warm clothes – for example, hat, scarf, gloves (fur-rimmed), jacket (with zip and buttons), boots and socks.
- Make a Guy Fawkes and feel the materials used in making him.
- Feel sticks and dried leaves.

Movement

- Encourage people to reach out to feel the different textures.
- Suggest people try on the different items.
- Encourage people to reach out and operate the switch for the fibre-optic spray (representing the bonfire). Create the 'bonfire' by putting red, orange and yellow cellophane over the fibre-optic spray and feel that as well.

Seeing

- Create 'stars' by making holes in blue acetate. Place on the overhead projector and project onto wall/ceiling.

Hearing

- Play sounds of fireworks, fire burning.

Smell

- Light sparklers outside – watch the sparklers and smell the smoke when they have burnt out. If anyone has a wood fire, let the smoke from the fire drift onto the clothes. Smell the wood smoke.

Taste

- Make and sample hot chocolate and toffee apples.

    Copyright © Scope (Vic.) Ltd 2008

FIREWORK DISPLAY

Equipment required

- Fan
- Ice bricks from the freezer
- Frozen ice pops
- Woolly hats and scarves
- Catherine wheel
- Coloured gels

- Sparklers
- Tape-recorder
- BIGMacks™
- Ingredients for making hot chocolate, popcorn, different herbal teas or coffee

How to use the story/theme to stimulate the different senses

Touch

- Cold windy night – use fan to create wind on people's faces.
- Feel ice bricks from the freezer (plastic containers with water inside, used to keep lunch bags cool). *Do not* use straight from the freezer because they will be too cold and will stick to people's skin.
- Feel frozen ice pops.
- Feel woolly hats and scarves.

Movement

- Encourage people to reach out and feel the different textures.
- Encourage people to reach out and turn on the catherine wheel using the switch.

Seeing

- Watch the patterns from the catherine wheel.
- Make up a solar effects wheel with different coloured patterns (e.g. using the coloured gels for spotlights), or use the fireworks effects wheel.
- Use sparklers – outside the MSR.

Hearing

- Record popping sounds, whooshing sounds, etc. Encourage people to make their own sounds and record them onto BIGMacks™ that they can then operate themselves.

Smell

- Smell the fumes from the sparklers.

Taste

- In the kitchen, make hot chocolate, popcorn, different herbal teas or coffee made from beans.

Copyright © Scope (Vic.) Ltd 2008

DISCO PARTY

Equipment required

- Different types of party clothes
- UV lamp
- Mirror ball
- Spotlight
- Sound system
- Essential oils
- Ingredients for different types of drinks

How to use the story/theme to stimulate the different senses

Touch

- Feel different types of party clothes – for example, feather boa, fur-rimmed gloves, brocade jacket, sequined pants, lace jacket, velvet pants, etc.

Movement

- Try on the clothing.
- Encourage people to reach out to feel the white items displayed under UV light.
- Dance and move to the music.

Seeing

- Use the mirror ball and spotlight as a disco ball.
- Look at white objects under UV light.

Hearing

- Listen to different types of music.

Smell

- Smell invigorating oils – for example, peppermint.

Taste

- Make up different types of drinks to try in the kitchen – for example, fruit smoothies, fruit cocktails.

 Copyright © Scope (Vic.) Ltd 2008

ALI BABA AND THE 40 THIEVES

Ali Baba was a poor man who made money by cutting and selling wood. One day in the forest he spotted a band of robbers and climbed a tree to hide from them. Ali Baba was up the tree for a long time while the robbers had a party with belly dancers and plenty of wine and food. When the party ended and the belly dancers had gone, Ali Baba heard the robbers approach a shrub and say 'Open Sesame', after which a door opened and the robbers disappeared. After they had gone, he went to the shrub, said the same words and a door opened up in a rock behind it. He walked inside and found a huge cave filled with treasure.

Later, when the thieves found that someone had taken some of their treasure, they found out where Ali Baba lived. They hid in terracotta jars of oil to gain entrance to his house and they were going to attack him in the night. Fortunately, a maid found out about the plan and Ali Baba was saved.

Equipment required

- Chiffon and gold coin scarves
- Rope lights
- Red/yellow cellophane
- Middle Eastern music
- Jewellery
- Coloured glass/Stones/Marbles
- Mesh bag
- Gold coloured plates, jugs, etc. to represent treasure
- Terracotta pots
- Bark and leaves from tree
- Fibre-optic spray
- Sound system
- Turkish Delight and Baklava ingredients
- Hummus ingredients

How to use the story/theme to stimulate the different senses

Touch

- Jewellery, coloured glass/stones/marbles. Keep these in a mesh bag if people are liable to put them in their mouth. Gold coloured plates, jugs, etc. (treasure).
- Terracotta pots.
- Chiffon scarves, gold coin scarves – for the belly dancer.
- Feel bark from a tree.
- Feel leaves dried and fresh.

Movement

- Someone to do a belly dance.
- Encourage people to reach out to touch the scarves moving on the belly dancer.

Seeing

- Use rope lights to outline a doorway or entrance to a tent to represent going into a cave or grotto.
- Use the fibre-optic spray with red/yellow cellophane to represent the fire the dancer moves around.

Hearing

- Middle Eastern music.
- Listen to the bells on the belly dancer.

Smell

- Smell Turkish Delight.

Taste

- Make Turkish Delight, Baklava (be aware that Baklava has nuts and may not be suitable for people with swallowing difficulties). Make and taste hummus.

 Copyright © Scope (Vic.) Ltd 2008

CREATE A CAVE ENVIRONMENT

Create a mini cave environment in a corner of a room or in a small tent.

Equipment required

- Large cardboard cylinders
- Papier mâché
- Art materials for making fur bat
- Rocks
- Lilo
- Black sheet
- Fluorescent paint
- Lace netting

- Fairy lights
- Black cloth
- Fibre-optic spray
- Torches
- Sound system
- Fresh mud, moss
- Cold drinks

How to use the story/theme to stimulate the different senses

Touch

- Cover large cardboard cylinders with papier mâché to make stalactites. Let the paper bunch up to give a rough texture.
- Make up fur bats to suspend in the cave.
- Find some rocks and feel their different textures and coldness.

Movement

- People to sit/lie on a lilo covered with a black sheet. Rock gently on the lilo to represent a raft in an underwater cave.

Seeing

- Paint the stalactites with fluorescent paint.
- Paint on lace netting with fluorescent paint and suspend in the cave.
- Hang up fairy lights or sew them onto black cloth (for glow worms).
- Use the fibre-optic spray to represent glow worms in the cave.
- Shine torches around the room.

Hearing

- Listen to sounds of water, bats, echoes.

Smell

- Smell fresh mud, moss.

Taste

- Make up cold drinks to taste.

THE NIGHT SKY, OR THE STORY OF ORION THE HUNTER

Set up a dark environment for people to explore, or use it as a setting for a story. For example, tell the story of Orion. Orion is a hunter who hunts Taurus the Bull with his dogs Canis Major and Canis Minor. He is in love with a princess but is not allowed to marry her. He becomes enraged and harms Metrope, the princess. He is punished by being blinded and cast into a deep sleep. To regain his sight, he has to travel east and let the rays of sunlight strike his eyes. After regaining his sight, he goes to live in Crete, where Artemis the goddess of the moon falls in love with him. One day he is swimming in the ocean and is accidentally killed with an arrow from Artemis' bow. As a consequence, the goddess places Orion in the sky with his dogs as the mightiest hunters of the night sky.

Equipment required

- Black material
- Metal belt or buckle
- Fur
- Tiara
- Silk material
- Survival blanket
- Water spray

- Glittery paper and art materials
- Effects wheel
- Fairy lights
- Torch
- Lamp, power box, switch
- Garlic and Mediterranean fruits

How to use the story/theme to stimulate the different senses

Touch

- Provide different textures of black material to feel.
- Feel a metal belt or belt buckle (Orion's belt).
- Stroke fur to represent the dogs.
- Feel a tiara and silk material belonging to the princess.
- Feel a survival blanket.
- Feel water from a water spray to represent the ocean.

Movement

- Encourage people to reach out and feel the different textures.

Seeing

- Make up a mobile of moons and planets using glittery paper.
- Make up an effects wheel with stars and planets.
- Suspend fairy lights above thin black material to represent the stars.
- Use a torch to represent stars.
- Make up an effects wheel with the constellations of Orion, Taurus and Canis Major and Minor.
- Link a lamp to a power box and use a switch to turn on the lamp. Direct the light onto a survival blanket to represent the rays of the sun.

 Copyright © Scope (Vic.) Ltd 2008

Hearing

- Listen to the sounds of the survival blanket when scrunched.

Smell

- Smell garlic, stuffed olives.

Taste

- Mediterranean fruits – for example, grapes, olives, grape juice; garlic.

A TRIP TO OUTER SPACE

Equipment required

- Papier mâché/paper pulp
- Art materials to make alien puppets/finger puppets
- Infinity tunnel
- Fluorescent paper/paint
- Silver foil/survival blanket
- Holographic paper

- BIGMacks™
- Soundbeam
- Powdered orange juice
- Swiss cheese
- 'Astronaut' rations such as chocolate and milk powder

How to use the story/theme to stimulate the different senses

Touch

- Make up planets, rockets, etc. using papier mâché/paper pulp. Leave some of the surfaces rough to add texture.
- Make alien puppets/finger puppets.

Movement

- Encourage people to reach out and feel the different textures.
- Encourage people to reach out and turn on the infinity tunnel using the switch.

Seeing

- Use the infinity tunnel to represent the Milky Way.
- Make up a mobile of moons and planets using fluorescent paper/paint.
- Cover the rocket with silver foil/survival blanket or holographic paper.
- Use alien puppets behind a projection screen so that people can watch the shadows.

Hearing

- Record messages from the 'astronauts' on BIGMacks™.
- Use the galaxy sounds from the Soundbeam.
- Listen to the sounds make by crumpling the foil/survival blanket.

Smell

- Smell the 'astronaut' rations and orange juice.

Taste

- Make up 'astronaut' rations to take on the space ship – for example, chocolate, vanilla mousse, milk powder.
- Make up orange juice using powdered orange juice.
- Taste Swiss cheese with holes in it.

Copyright © Scope (Vic.) Ltd 2008

GO FOR A JOURNEY THROUGH OUTER SPACE

Set the scene with the astronauts getting ready to blast off in their rocket. Look for music about space and blasting off – for example, 'Silver Balloon (1995) by Paul Jamieson'. This has a countdown from ten before blasting off. Set up an experience of travelling in a rocket and passing different planets, satellites and space stations. Arrive at a space station for lunch.

Equipment required

- Art materials to make collages and mobiles
- Papier mâché ingredients
- Bubble wrap
- Baking tray
- Chicken wire
- Mosquito netting
- Cornflour and water
- Coloured dough ingredients
- Glow-in-the-dark stars
- UV lamp
- Cotton wool
- Lace

- Peppermint, ginger
- Ingredients for making peppermint creams and ginger biscuits
- Leaf chair
- Hammock
- Vibroacoustic
- Survival blanket
- Sound system
- Old spoons and forks
- Different cheeses
- Projector

How to use the story/theme to stimulate the different senses

Touch

- Make up a 'junk' collage of satellites and space stations, exploring the properties of the different cartons, plastic, cardboard tubes. Make textured papier mâché planets, planet mobiles, rockets, etc. When making papier mâché, place bubble wrap on the bottom of a baking tray. Make flour, salt and water glue using warm water. Place pieces of paper in the baking tray and encourage people to coat the paper in glue with their hands. Place different textures on the bottom of the tray – for example, chicken wire, mosquito netting – so that people can experience touching different textures while coating the paper in glue (Leanne Crawford).

- Moon craters can be made from mixing cornflour and water, or make coloured dough and use this to model objects for the deep space theme.

Movement

- Sit/lie in a leaf chair, hammock, vibroacoustic beanbag or vibrating mat, put lace over it and project a picture of a rocket to represent sitting in a rocket.

Copyright © Scope (Vic.) Ltd 2008

✓

Seeing

- Use glow-in-the-dark stars and create a space theme with glittery and fluorescent mobiles of stars, planets and spaceships. Also use black and white items and cotton wool clouds to be highlighted under UV light. Take a slide photo of the collage under UV light and project it onto different surfaces – for example, lace curtain, survival blanket.
- Paint the junk collage in silver paint or cover with tinfoil.

Hearing

- Play cassettes/CDs – for example, *The Planets* by Holst.
- Make up a planet wind chime by placing a wire hoop around a papier mâché planet and suspend old spoons and forks to represent stars/moons around the planet.

Smell

- Smell peppermint, ginger (travel sickness!); could be anything – we don't know about smells in outer space!

Taste

- Make peppermint creams, ginger biscuits and link smell and taste.
- Try different cheeses (the moon is made of cheese!).

Copyright © Scope (Vic.) Ltd 2008

A VISIT TO THE PUB

Use this outline to recount a person's own visit to the pub.

Equipment required

- Different fabrics and materials to represent chairs of the pub and clothes worn
- Vibrating mat
- Leaf chair
- Ladder light
- Sound system
- Ginger
- Crisps/nuts
- Ingredients to make beer/ginger beer

How to use the story/theme to stimulate the different senses

Touch

- Feel different fabrics for the chairs.
- Feel different materials (for clothes worn to the pub).
- Sit on the vibrating mat to represent the trip in the car to the pub.

Movement

- Sit in the leaf chair to represent the trip in the car to the pub.

Seeing

- Sing along to the music or watch the lights on the ladder light change with the music (karaoke).

Hearing

- Play music.
- Record people talking and experiment with the volume. Make it louder as more people come to the pub.

Smell

- Smell ginger used to make ginger beer.

Taste

- Make and taste beer/ginger beer.
- Nibble crisps/nuts (ensure that people are safe to eat these foods).

SET UP A RELAXING ENVIRONMENT WITH A VISIT TO A SPA

Equipment required

- Footspa
- Warm fluffy towels
- Peppermint foot balm
- Projector
- Sound system
- Scented products for the footspa

How to use the story/theme to stimulate the different senses

Touch

- Sit with feet in the footspa.
- Dry feet with warm fluffy towels.
- Massage peppermint foot lotion into the feet.

Movement

- Sit in a leaf chair or hammock after a foot spa, and watch the images on the wall from there.

Seeing

- Dim the lights and project an image onto the wall for people to look at.

Hearing

- Play relaxing music. Use different types of music to find out which people find most relaxing.

Smell

- Use scented products in the footspa.

Taste

- Finish the activity by eating a piece of chocolate or chocolate mousse (or alternative comfort food).

 Copyright © Scope (Vic.) Ltd 2008

SET UP A RELAXING ENVIRONMENT WITH THE VIBRATING BED OR MASSAGE MAT

Equipment required

- Vibrating bed
- Massage mat
- Projector

- Fibre-optic spray
- Sound system
- Relaxing oils

How to use the story/theme to stimulate the different senses

Touch

- Sit/lie on the vibrating bed on a low setting, or sit/lie on a massage mat.

Movement

- Sit in a leaf chair or hammock.

Seeing

- Project an image onto the wall for people to look at, or drape the fibre-optic spray around them on the bed.

Hearing

- Play relaxing music. Use different types of music to find out which creates the most relaxing environment for people.

Smell

- Blow the aroma of relaxing oils into the room.

Taste

- Finish the activity by eating a piece of chocolate or chocolate mousse (or alternative comfort food).

CREATE AN ATMOSPHERE FOR A MULTISENSORY MASSAGE

Equipment required

- Lotions/oils/powders
- Different materials to massage with
- Solar projector
- Coloured disco light gels
- Sound system
- Aromatherapy diffuser
- Scented plugs

How to use the story/theme to stimulate the different senses

Touch

- Use different types of lotions/oils/powders for a massage.
- Use different types of material to massage with – for example, fur, silk, cord.
- Use different types of massage devices – for example, 'massage dolphin', wooden bead massager, hand-held electric massager.

Movement

- Sit in a leaf chair or hammock.

Seeing

- Project the liquid wheel from the solar projector onto the wall.
- Make up a colour wheel using coloured disco light gels.

Hearing

- Listen to relaxing music.

Smell

- Smell the aroma from an aromatherapy diffuser – for example, lavender. Plugs for the wall are also available, which have bottles of lavender essential oil to diffuse.

Taste

- Finish the activity by eating a piece of chocolate or chocolate mousse (or alternative comfort food).

 Copyright © Scope (Vic.) Ltd 2008

RECREATE AN EVENT THAT PEOPLE HAVE ATTENDED SUCH AS A FOOTIE MATCH

Take photographs and use with a slide projector or computer to recount the story.

Equipment required

- Slide projector or computer
- Footie jumper, beanie and scarf
- Footie streamers
- Sound system
- Tape-recorder
- Creams and spray for sore muscles
- Footie food and drink such as pies and lemonade

How to use the story/theme to stimulate the different senses

Touch

- Feel the fabrics of a footie jumper, beanie and scarf.

Movement

- Encourage people to reach out to feel the different textures and operate the switch to change the pictures.
- Shake footie streamers.

Seeing

- Show slides that have been taken at the footie match.
- Use a switch to change the pictures on the slide projector or computer.

Hearing

- Play the theme song of the teams you went to watch. Play the sound of the crowd recorded at the footie match.

Smell

- Smell 'deep heat' and other creams used on sore muscles.

Taste

- Taste a pie at the footie match. Drink lemonade.

VOLCANO THEME

Equipment required

- Hammock
- Vibroacoustic beanbag
- Leaf chair
- Vibrating mat
- Rocks

- Data projector and computer
- Red and yellow lights
- Sound system
- Smoky jumper and such like

How to use the story/theme to stimulate the different senses

Touch

- Feel warm rocks and compare with cold rocks.
- Feel the different textures of rocks.

Movement

- Lie in a hammock, on a vibroacoustic beanbag, leaf chair or vibrating mat to represent the ground shaking from the volcano erupting.

Seeing

- Use a data projector and computer to project images of volcanoes erupting.
- Watch red and yellow lights flicking on and off.
- Turn off the lights and experience being in darkness.

Hearing

- Listen to the roar of volcanoes erupting.
- Listen to the sound of rocks falling.

Smell

- Smell of smoke (maybe from a jumper worn when standing around a bonfire).

Taste

- Taste a hot drink e.g. hot chocolate, coffee, malt, etc.

 Copyright © Scope (Vic.) Ltd 2008

THE BEACH THEME

Equipment required

- Marine animals such as fish and octopus
- Beach material such as sand, shells and seaweed
- Papier mâché
- Bathing clothes
- Fibre-optic cave
- Fan
- Heat pack
- Leaf chair
- Hammock
- Vibrating mat
- Art materials to make prints, mobiles and kites
- Cellophane to make seaweed
- Sound system
- Bubble tube
- Glass fish
- Solar projector
- Blue cloth
- Survival blanket
- Umbrella
- Aromatherapy diffuser
- Coconut sun lotion
- Ingredients for coconut ice
- Salt
- Water/juice
- Fish and chips
- Ice-cream

How to use the story/theme to stimulate the different senses

Touch

- Feel tactile fish, octopus, sand, shells, seaweed, fish prints in art, papier mâché people lying on the beach, cloth bathers, objects in the fibre-optic cave (sheltering from the sun), wind from a fan, heat pack.

Movement

- Swing in a leaf chair (or hammock), lie on a vibrating mat (getting a massage on the beach). Set up objects that encourage people to want to reach out and move their arms – for example, make 'beach mobiles' with sand, sandpaper with cinnamon, silver paper.

Seeing

- Watch bubbles moving in the bubble tube (put glass fish in).
- Use the solar projector with a surfer projected onto blue cloth.
- Represent the sun by projecting light onto a survival blanket (glare of sun) or project yellow light for the sun.
- Project beach images onto an umbrella (sunshade).
- Decorate room with fish prints.
- Pass around a heated wheat pack or turn up the heating!
- Make fish mobiles.
- Make kites or use plain kites and project beach images onto them.

Copyright © Scope (Vic.) Ltd 2008

Hearing

- Crumple the cellophane seaweed, listen to the sound of waves, dolphins, wind from a fan, seagulls, beach songs (e.g. by the Beachboys).

Smell

- Use an aromatherapy diffuser with beach smells – for example, coconut. Use electric or fan-forced aromatherapy diffusers, not candles.
- Smell coconut sun lotion, seaweed.

Taste

- Make coconut ice, taste salt, water/juice, buy fish and chips, ice-cream.

Copyright © Scope (Vic.) Ltd 2008

ARABIAN NIGHTS THEME

Equipment required

- Chiffon scarves
- Lace
- Sand
- Sultan's hat
- Small pool of water
- Fan
- Leaf chair
- Projector

- Coloured cellophane
- Fibre optics
- Glow-in-the-dark stars
- Sound system
- Fire
- Animal dung
- Middle Eastern food
- Ingredients to make Turkish Delight and Baklava

How to use the story/theme to stimulate the different senses

Touch

- Feel chiffon scarves, lace, sand, sultan's hat, oasis (small pool of water – may need to be explored outside the room).
- Feel wind from a fan and direct it onto chiffon scarves hanging as curtains.

Movement

- Find people to do a belly dance!!
- Sit in a leaf chair (sultan lying on the divan, or riding a camel).

Seeing

- Project pictures of camels, belly dancers, sand dunes, oases.
- Make a fire with coloured cellophane over the fibre-optics.
- Look at glow-in-the-dark stars (open sky in the desert).

Hearing

- Listen to bells, camel noises, Middle Eastern music, fire.

Smell

- Fire, animal dung! Middle Eastern food.

Taste

- Make Turkish Delight. For those who can eat nuts, make/buy Baklava.

Copyright © Scope (Vic.) Ltd 2008

LEAF THEME

Equipment required

- Leaves
- Box
- Leaf mobile
- Leaf chair
- Netting
- Materials to make leaf wheels
- Projector
- Fan
- Tape-recorder
- Power box
- Herbs
- Eucalyptus leaves
- Pine-scented car fresheners
- Edible leaves

How to use the story/theme to stimulate the different senses

Touch

- Feel dried leaves in a box.

Movement

- Hang a leaf mobile over a leaf chair, hang netting over the leaf chair and attach leaves to it.

Seeing

- Make leaf wheels to project using real leaves, leaf silhouettes, clip art, photos or drawings of leaves. Project pictures of different types of trees.

Hearing

- Listen to dried leaves in a box, wind from a fan on dried leaves, wind in trees on a tape (make the session interactive by plugging the tape-recorder into a power box and encouraging people to turn on the tape-recorder).

Smell

- Smell herbs, eucalyptus leaves, car fresheners – pine-scented. Integrate with other sessions – for example, collect lavender from a garden or gardening centre.

Taste

- Think about other leaves in the environment and taste them – for example, tea leaves. Taste different types of leaves – for example, camomile/peppermint teas, spinach pie, lettuce and herb scones.

 Copyright © Scope (Vic.) Ltd 2008

Useful organizations

Abilitations Multisensory
PO Box 922668
Norcross
GA 30010–2668
USA
Tel: 770 449 5700
Fax: 770 510 7290
Website: www.abilitation.com

Indomed Pty Ltd
41 Forsyth St
O'Connor
WA 6163
Australia
Tel: 0061 (08) 9331 6711
Fax: 0061 (08) 9331 672
Email: indomed@iinet.net.au
Website: www.indomed.com.au

Kirton Playworks
The Printworks
Sealand Road
Chester CH1 4QS
UK
Tel: 0044 (0) 1244 399731
Fax: 0044 (0) 1244 398206
Website: www.kirtonplayworks.com

Mike Ayres Design and Development Ltd
The Paddocks
Dore
Sheffield S17 3LD
UK
Tel: 0044 (0) 113 235 6880
Fax: 0044 (0) 114 235 6881
Email: enquiry@mike-ayres.co.uk
Website: www.mike-ayres.co.uk

Copyright © Scope (Vic.) Ltd 2008

ROMPA

Goyt Side Road
Chesterfield
Derbyshire S40 2PH
UK
Tel: 0044 (0) 1246 211777
Fax: 0044 (0) 1246 221802
Website: www.rompa.com

Sensco Multisensory Environments

114 Bentinck House
Bentinck Street
Ashton OL6 7SZ
UK
Tel: 0044 (0) 161 343 8823
Email: enquiries@sensco.co.uk
Website: www.sensco.co.uk

Soundbeam Project

Unit 3, Highbury Villas
St Michaels Hill
Bristol
BS2 8BY
UK
Tel: 0044 (0)117 974 4142
Fax: 0044 (0)117 970 6241
Email: tim@soundbeam.co.uk

Spacekraft Ltd

Titus House
29 Saltaire road
Shipley
West Yorkshire BD18 3HH
UK
Tel: 0044 (0) 1274 581007
Fax: 0044 (0) 1274 531966
Website: www.spacekraft.co.uk

Technical Solutions

109 Ferndale Road
Silvan
Vic 3795
Australia
Tel: 0061 (03) 9739 9000
Fax: 0061 (03) 9737 9111

Copyright © Scope (Vic.) Ltd 2008

The Sensory Company International Ltd
Broad Lane Business Centre
Westfield Lane
South Elmsall WF9 2JX
UK
Tel: 0044 (0) 845 838 2233
Fax: 0044 (0) 845 838 2234
Website: www.thesensorycompany.co.uk

Wilkins Inernational Pty Ltd
H Unit 14 173–181 Rooks Road,
Vermont 3133
Australia
Tel: 0061 (03) 9874 1033
Fax: 0061 (03) 9874 6611
Website: www.wilkinsinternational.com.au

Copyright © Scope (Vic.) Ltd 2008

✓

Community sensory activities

Touch activities

- Outside – physically explore, e.g. bark of trees, brick walls, fences, plants and flowers, etc.

- Explore the textures of materials and haberdashery

- Explore textures at hardware stores, e.g. plastic grating

- Horse riding – grooming the horse

- Visiting farms and stroking the animals

- Pet therapy

- Community art centres and neighbourhood houses offer a variety of activities, e.g. ceramics, painting, collage activities, cookery

- Visit beautician for facials, having nails done

- Visit masseur/aromatherapist

- Beauty care/perfume counters (touch and smell)

- Hairdresser – find one that also offers a head massage

- Bead car seat covers for the car

- Ball pools

Movement activities

NB. Please take care with these movement-based activities. Consult with a therapist before swivelling people around as it can make them sick and could cause seizures.

- Trampoline activities

- Swing activities

- Slides

- Roundabouts in playgrounds

- Inflatables at fêtes

- Hammock activities

- Seesaw activities

 Copyright © Scope (Vic.) Ltd 2008

- Rocking chair

- Lying on an airbed

- Leaf chair (obtained through companies who provide multisensory equipment.

- Children's soft play areas

- Executive swivel chairs

- Wheelchair/bush dancing in community/leisure centres

- Walks along the beach over different surfaces (in the wheelchair)

- Being pushed in a wheelchair over a rough surface

- Being pushed in a wheelchair along a pier

- Swimming

- Jacuzzi/spa

- Wave pool

- Sailing

- Horse riding

- Ice skating (skating whilst pushing wheelchairs on the ice)

- Music and movement sessions at neighbourhood houses, community centres, leisure centres

- Moving through the Soundbeam used in community electronic music programmes

- Feldenkrais – movement awareness programme

- Lying/seating on a wobbleboard

- Taking a train ride – stopping at all stations

- Going on the bus, in a car

- Taking a boat ride

- Riding in a lift

- Being in the hoist

Seeing activities

- Aquarium

- Art galleries and museums

- Firework displays

Copyright © Scope (Vic.) Ltd 2008

✓

- Imax – 3D cinemas
- Jewellery counters
- Shops selling holograms and holographic paper
- Christmas lights in streets and shops
- Blow some bubbles in the park
- Feeding the seagulls (also auditory)

Hearing activities

- Record shops – try the listening posts if people can tolerate headphones
- Concerts
- Pub bands
- Football matches
- Railway station
- Church
- Music shops with musical instruments
- Some playgrounds and gardens have sound sculptures and sound-making equipment

Smell/olfactory activities

- Perfume counters
- Body Shop/Red Earth
- Visiting an aromatherapist
- Herb gardens
- Sensory gardens
- Botanical gardens
- Farms
- Bakery
- Restaurants
- Pet shops
- Fish shop
- Market

Copyright © Scope (Vic.) Ltd 2008

Taste activities

- Restaurants
- Cafes
- Pub food
- Ice-cream parlours
- Bakers
- Dairies/cheese farms
- Wine tasting
- Chocolate tasting

Mandy Williams and Susan Fowler (2001)

Copyright © Scope (Vic.) Ltd 2008

Sensory banks

Flo Longhorn described the concept of sensory banks in her book *A Sensory Curriculum for Very Special People* (1988). They are collections of different types of materials and equipment, *categorized according to the different senses.* For example: an auditory bank could contain objects, which make sounds, e.g. wind chimes, musical instruments and paper that rustles when crunched; a visual bank could have items that encourage people to look and track and could include torches, tinsel and, silver paper that glitters; and a tactile bank could include a collection of tactile materials with different properties, e.g. hard, soft, furry, rough, crinkly, sticky. It could also include items that vibrate. Vibration is such a powerful tactile/movement stimulus that vibrating tactile banks can be set up as a bank in their own right. This could include vibrating keyrings, hand-held massagers, footspas, vibrating mats, seats and cushions, vibrating hairbrushes – the list is endless.

Sensory banks are a useful way to store materials for use in creating *individual multisensory environments.* If a person is very motivated by tactile objects, the tactile bank can be used as a resource to find objects that will interest that person. These objects can then be mounted on a frame and suspended around a person to create their own mini tactile environment. Alternatively, activity arches can be set up which are *theme based.* The equipment from each theme could be stored together; for example, bathroom equipment, kitchen equipment and gardening equipment.

The materials in the sensory banks can also be used for *sensory activities.* Thus a tactile collage could be made from the materials in the tactile bank, which may include different types of pasta, beans and rice. Obviously some of the categories overlap so that the pasta, beans and rice could also be used for an auditory session, if they were placed inside sealed tubes and tipped from one end to the other.

Sensory banks are a useful resource if you want to plan *sensory theme rooms* or corners. People can be involved in creating their own sensory environments such as an underwater corner or deep space room. These sensory environments can be planned as a long-term project. For example, one week people could explore the properties of the different types of paper used for the weeds, water, etc. The next week the properties of different textures, used to make sea creatures such as fish, octopus or seahorses, could be explored. Another week people could visit the beach and collect sand and shells for the room. Once the room is ready, a fan with a power box and switch could be set up so that people can make the 'seaweed' move.

Not only can sensory banks be a way to store resources but they can be used as an *assessment tool* as well. Equipment from the various banks can be used to see what exactly motivates a person to explore. Those same pieces of equipment can then be brought and put in a bag or box for the sole use of that person. This also addresses the hygiene

Copyright © Scope (Vic.) Ltd 2008

issue of different people using the different pieces of equipment. People must be rigorous in keeping the pieces of equipment in the sensory banks disinfected.

It is important not to clutter a room because it can be visually over-stimulating and difficult to manoeuvre through. It is therefore preferable to keep equipment in sensory banks either outside the room or shut away in a cupboard until required.

Equipment checklist for sensory equipment

Use this form to help decide whether or not a piece of equipment is suitable for your needs.

Name of equipment	
Which sensory system(s) does this piece of equipment stimulate?	
What are people's needs? (specify)	
Touch	
Movement	
Seeing	
Hearing	
Smell	
Taste	
How many different ways can you use this piece of equipment?	
Assessment	
Skills development: • Hand–eye co-ordination • Cause and effect • Switch use • Cognitive skills • Visual tracking/stimulation • Auditory tracking/stimulation • Tactile stimulation	

Copyright © Scope (Vic.) Ltd 2008

Functional skills	
Communication skills	
Person engagement	
Object engagement	
Person–object engagement	
Relaxation	
Leisure	
Theme work	

Does this piece of equipment meet people's needs?	
How much does the equipment cost?	
Who supplies this piece of equipment?	
Do you think this piece of equipment has enough different uses to merit the cost?	
Do you need this equipment to be adapted so that it is more suitable for the people you support? Who could do this?	
Could you make/buy a similar piece of equipment that is cheaper?	
Signature:	Date:

Copyright © Scope (Vic.) Ltd 2008

Multisensory environments equipment analysis

Use this form for a more in-depth analysis of the equipment you are using.

Name of equipment	
What senses does the equipment stimulate?	
Touch	
Movement	
Seeing	
Hearing	
Smell	
Taste	
What can you assess with this piece of equipment?	
How can you use the equipment to encourage the development of skills?	
How can you use the equipment to encourage relaxation?	
How can you use the equipment for leisure (e.g. theme work/stories)?	

 Copyright © Scope (Vic.) Ltd 2008

Below is an example of equipment analysis.

Name of equipment:

Bubble tube.

What senses does the equipment stimulate?

Touch

Feels hard/cool, feel the vibrations from the pump.

Movement

Move hands around the tube.

Seeing

Watch the bubbles moving, changing colours.

Hearing

Listen to the sound of the pump humming.

Smell

Not applicable.

Taste

Not applicable.

What can you assess with this piece of equipment?

- Engagement behaviours.

- Sensory preferences.

- Visual skills – visual location, ability to sustain fixation and visual tracking.

- Hearing skills – ability to hear and locate hum of bubble tube.

- Communication skills.

- Cognitive skills.

- Switching skills.

- Motivation for using this piece of equipment – like, dislike, disinterest.

How can you use the equipment to encourage the development of skills

Engagement behaviours and sensory preferences

- Do people exhibit self-engagement behaviours? What are they?

- Do people stop self-engagement behaviours when interacting with the bubble tube?

- What sensory aspects of the bubble tube result in people stopping or reducing self-engagement behaviours?

- How do people interact with the bubble tube?

  ○ Do people like the feel of the bubble tube when off? (E.g. do they like the hard, smooth texture?)

  ○ Do they like the bubble tube when it comes on (no colours)? (E.g. like the vibrations?)

  ○ Are they more interested watching the changing colours of bubbles?

  ○ Are they more interested in listening to the hum of the pump?

Tactile stimulation

- Do people pull away when touched with the equipment (e.g. switch for bubble tube or bubble tube itself)

- Do people let the equipment/switch rest in/on their hand?

- Do people actively feel the equipment/switch? (If not, help them by moving the equipment across the hand and/or closing their hands around the equipment and gently squeezing their hand so that they can feel the object inside.)

- Help people to reach forward to feel the vibrations from the bubble column. Do they like to feel the vibrations from the bubble tube either with their hands, foot or full body? Specify.

- Do people reach for the equipment/switch independently?

Visual stimulation

- Do people notice when the bubble tube comes on and turn to look (e.g. notices change in the environment)?

- Do people look fleetingly then look away?

- Do people look for a sustained period of time? (How long?)

- Do people look if they are near the bubble tube?

- Do people look if they are far away from the bubble tube?

- How near do they have to be before they notice the bubbles and colours?

 Copyright © Scope (Vic.) Ltd 2008

- Do people watch (track) the bubbles moving in the column? (Remember the equipment will have to gain their attention before they can track. If the bubbles are moving too quickly it may be difficult for the person to track them.)

- Do people track from side to side?

- Do people track up and down?

- Do people track as the bubbles move randomly?

- Do they notice when the colours change?

- Do they notice the different colours?

Auditory stimulation

- Turn people away so they cannot see the bubble tube – do they react when the pump is turned on?

- Do people look towards the source of the sound?

- Do people show a fleeting interest in the sound or a sustained interest? (How long?)

- Do people like to put their ear to the bubble tube to hear the gurgling of the water?

Further questions to consider for auditory stimulation

- Do people notice when the equipment comes on (e.g. notices change in the environment)?

- Do people respond to particular types of music? (Which types? E.g. classical, hard rock, folk, pop, Chinese, Irish)

- Do people respond to particular musical instruments? (Which ones?)

- Do people react to a certain volume of sound (quiet/loud)?

- Do people respond to a certain pitch of sound?

- Do people respond to a certain rhythm of sound?

Olfactory stimulation

(Not relevant for the bubble tube but questions to consider.)

- Do people respond to different smells? How do they respond?

- What sort of smells do people like? How do they indicate this?

- Do certain smells help people to become more alert?

- Do certain smells help people to become more relaxed?

✓

- Do certain smells have certain associations for people (e.g. the smell of orange essential oil makes them think of oranges they can eat)?

Gustatory stimulation

- The sense of taste tends not to occur in MSRs, except in sensory gardens when tasting fruits, vegetables or herbs. It is more normal to present this type of stimuli during activities such as sensory cookery.

Person engagement behaviours (important for developing communication skills)

- Do people respond to you reproducing their vocalizations or movements? How?

- Do people react to name being called (e.g. turns head, opens eyes, smiles)?

- Do people give eye contact?

- Do people look at people momentarily?

- Do people look closely at another person's face?

- Do people watch a person moving around the room?

- Do people move away when you touch them in greeting?

- Do people passively greet you (e.g. leave their hand in yours)?

- Do people initiate contact (e.g. reach out to you)?

- Do people interact with their peers? (e.g. initiate and interact with them, share an object or activity with them)?

- Do people work co-operatively (e.g. one person operates the switch for bubbles on the bubble tube and the other operates the switch for colours)?

Communication skills

- Is there a change in a person's vocalizations when greeted or shown a piece of equipment?

- When noting if a person responds to a piece of equipment, document how they respond and what that means. For example, do people indicate an interest in the bubble tube by smiling, vocalizing?

- Do people try to get your attention? (How?)

- Do people make a choice between using the bubble tube and another piece of equipment? How do they make a choice?

- Do people recognize the object symbol, photograph, pictograph of the bubble tube?

Copyright © Scope (Vic.) Ltd 2008

- Do people share an interest in the bubble tube with you (e.g. looking at the bubble tube and looking at you)?

- Do people interact with you to indicate that they would like 'more' of the bubbles (put the bubble tube on a timer so that they have to interact with you to have it turned back on)?

Cognitive skills

- How long are people interested in looking, listening, feeling, before they lose interest? (attention span)

- Do people know cause and effect? For example, do they know that if they used the switch it will turn on the bubble tube?

- It is important to have the bubble tube on a timer if you want to keep people alert and teach them the concept of cause and effect. If the bubble tube is on all the time then there is no reason for people to use the switch. They can also habituate (get used) to the bubbles being on and they cease to be of interest.

- Do people match the colour of bubbles to the colour of the switch?

- Do people recognize the different colours?

- Do people anticipate an event (e.g. the changing colours of the bubbles or that they are going to the multisensory room)?

- Do people understand object permanence (e.g. knowing that something is still there even if they can't see it)? Hide the switches under little boxes or different pieces of fabric.

- Do people still locate the switches if they are partially hidden under a cloth/box?

- Assess memory – show people the switch, then hide it under a cloth. Do they remember where the switch is?

- Do people remember where the bubble tube is in the room? Are they able to take themselves to the bubble tube or look in the right direction?

- Do they remember how to turn the bubble tube on?

- Do people have numeracy skills? For example, can they count the number of coloured switches you use to operate the different colours in the bubble tube?

- Do people recognize body parts? For example, can they answer the question 'Is the switch by my leg or hand?'

- Do people understand concepts such as above, below, left, right (e.g. hold switch above the head, below the arm, to the left/right)?

Copyright © Scope (Vic.) Ltd 2008

- Do people recognize an object symbol for the MSR, or for a particular piece of equipment?

- Do people recognize the photograph or pictograph of the MSR or different pieces of equipment?

- Do people understand the concepts of 'on' and 'off'?

- Do people understand the concepts of 'up' and 'down'?

Switching skills

- Can people co-ordinate hand and eye/foot and eye to operate a switch?

- Are they using switches in a functional way to practise hand–eye co-ordination?

- Do people use the switch purposefully or accidentally?

- Do people understand that they have used the switch (i.e. have an understanding of cause and effect)?

- Do people take turns using the switch?

How can you use the equipment to encourage relaxation?

- Use the bubble tube as a focal point. Darken the room, play soft relaxing music, use relaxing aromas and ensure people are comfortable, either in a chair or on a mat.

How can you use the equipment for leisure (e.g. theme work/stories)?

- Centre piece for underwater theme.

- Use in story/production (e.g. *Moby Dick, Jonah and the Whale*).

- Use as setting to recount an outing (e.g. visit to the aquarium

- Set up a game, with different people in charge of the different coloured switches. Call out a colour and the person holding that coloured switch operates it to change the colours in the bubble tube.

Copyright © Scope (Vic.) Ltd 2008

Engagement background questionnaire

Person's name: ....

Questionnaire date: ....

Completed by: ....

Relation to person: ....

Introduction

This questionnaire has been devised to gather information on the engagement behaviours of a person. It should be completed by one who has known the person long enough in order to be familiar with his or her behaviours.

Consider the following statements in each of the sections and tick the appropriate space according to your personal judgement of the behaviours of the person.

There is a choice between three responses for each statement. Please be sure to fill in only one space for a response.

Please read the brief definitions of the response categories provided below before filling in the questionnaire.

All completed questionnaires will be treated with absolute confidentiality.

Definitions of response choices	
YES	This statement is fairly typical of the person and occurs often during the day
NO	This statement is not at all typical of the person and does not occur during the day
SOMETIMES	This statement is not typical of the person but occurs sporadically or some of the time

This questionnaire was devised by Karen Bunning (speech and language therapist) and has been adapted by Susan Fowler (occupational therapist), October 1999

Copyright © Scope (Vic.) Ltd 2008

Section A: Self-engagement behaviours

Descriptive statement	Yes	No	Sometimes	Sensory system
Person walks in ritualistic patterns, repetitively				
Person engages in rocking behaviour				
Person bounces up and down repetitively on feet or seat				
Person spins self around repetitively whilst standing				
Person sways head from side to side, repetitively				
Person performs ritualistic hand and arm gestures				
Person flicks fingers in front of eyes and face repetitively				
Person picks up scraps from floor and other surfaces				
Person manipulates objects in ritualistic way (e.g. spinning, twiddling)				
Person manipulates own clothing repetitively				
Person touches self repetitively				
Person utters bizarre, irrelevant verbalizations				
Person emits screams, not obviously related to distress				
Person makes repetitive non-speech sounds				
Person engages in anal/oral behaviour inappropriately				
Person masturbates in inappropriate/public places				
Person engages in self-injurious behaviour				

Copyright © Scope (Vic.) Ltd 2008

Section B: Person engagement behaviours

Descriptive statement	Yes	No	Sometimes
Person reacts to name being called (e.g. turns head, opens eyes, smiles) (specify)			
Person gives eye contact			
Person looks at others momentarily			
Person looks closely at another person's face			
Person watches you/tracks you moving around the room			
Person reacts to another person offering hand in greeting (e.g. ignores, looks, pulls self away, reaches out) (specify)			
Person shows a response in reaction to you reproducing their movement or vocalization			
Person reacts to being touched in greeting (e.g. tolerates touch, shakes hands, smiles, pulls hand away, becomes agitated) (specify)			
Person changes vocalizations when greeted (e.g. becomes quiet, vocalizations increase) (specify)			
Person initiates contact (e.g. reaches for/touches in social contact)			
Person tries to get your attention in other ways (e.g. calls out, bangs the table) (specify)			
Person responds to a command (e.g. give me)			
Person imitates the actions of a person (e.g. waves goodbye) (specify)			

Copyright © Scope (Vic.) Ltd 2008

Section C: Object engagement behaviours

Descriptive statement	Yes	No	Sometimes
Person attends to an object			
Person tracks object			
Person watches objects near and/or far (specify)			
Person holds/explores object when placed in hand			
Person actively explores objects (e.g. mouth/lick, shake, throw, drop, hold, manipulate, visually inspects, listens to) (specify)			
Person reaches to touch objects			
Person picks up objects without prompting			
Person uses object purposefully and functionally			
Person vocalizes when given an object			
Person vocalizes when drops/loses an object			
Person attends to object for less than 30 seconds			
Person attends to object for more than 30 seconds (specify)			
Person has preferred object(s) (specify)			
Person makes choices between two/more objects			
Person indicates like/dislike (specify object)			

    Copyright © Scope (Vic.) Ltd 2008

Section D: Person–object engagement behaviours

Descriptive statement	Yes	No	Sometimes
Person looks between person and object			
Person uses an object to get a need met (e.g. holds up cup for a drink)			
Person co-actively passes an object to another person			
Person gives object to another person independently			
Person joins in activity with another person			
Person shows activity or object to another person			
Person indicates to person a desired object/activity			

Copyright © Scope (Vic.) Ltd 2008

✓

Likes and dislikes list

Name:		Date:
Likes & Dislikes List		
Sensory System & Social	**Likes**	**Dislikes**
Social	•	•
Movement	•	•
Touch	•	•
Hearing	•	•
Seeing	•	•
Smell	•	•
Taste	•	•

Copyright © Scope (Vic.) Ltd 2008

Questions to ask

Movement

Being in sling, bus, lift, swimming, going for walks, hammock, trampoline, wheelchair dancing, wheelchair soccer, hanging head down.

Tactile

ADL: bath/shower, having hair washed/dried, getting dressed, teeth brushed, preference for particular type of clothing, massage/footspa, people touching hand/arm/shoulders to say hello, shoes on/off, being close to people.

Auditory

Music – preferences, environmental sounds, e.g. birds, vacuum cleaner, sounds they make. Hands over ears?

Visual

Responds to lights on/off, likes glittery things, bright colours/lights, candles/torches, UV environment, being in sun/shade.

Taste/smell

Foods liked/disliked – taste, temperature, texture; likes perfumes/aftershave, massage oils, gardens. Particular objects likes to chew?

Social

Likes being with other people/being alone? Enjoys one-to-one interactions. Responds to people mirroring vocalizations or movements.

Physical environment

Noisy, quiet, crowds, small groups, solitary, market, shopping centre, other.

Other

Anything else people like/dislike.

Copyright © Scope (Vic.) Ltd 2008

✓

Personal communication dictionary

Personal communication dictionary for: _____		
What _____ does (describe behaviours, when, where and what occurs)	**What this might mean (interpret the behaviour)**	**What you should do (how communication partner should respond)**

People involved in completing this form:

Date commenced:

Karen Bloomberg

Copyright © Scope (Vic.) Ltd 2008

Example of a sensory story – The park

Story Line	Equipment	Sounds – soundscape	Narrative – telling the story
Walk on a gravel path	Bowl with gravel	Listen to sounds of walking on gravel	Walking A path Crunching gravel
Walk over a bridge and look at the stream	Feel wood from bridge Look at fibre-optic spray Switch	Bridge sounds – walking over wooden bridge	We go over the bridge Wooden bridge Walking over water Water rushing, babbling Water swishing, running Underneath the bridge
Look at the water feature	Bubble tube Switch	Water sounds – a watery soundscape	Looking Moving water Babbling Swishing
Sitting in the sun (very hot)	Survival blanket with lamp to represent sun Sunblock Look at shadows – difference between light and dark	Summer sounds – crickets chirping	It's hot now, sitting In the sun A big round ball Colours in the light Light and dark Day and night

Story Line	Equipment	Sounds – soundscape	Narrative – telling the story
Sit in a forest	Forest netting on grid Paper pulp/material leaves Animals UV light Fan switch Eucalyptus leaves (or oil on leaves) Wet and dry grass clippings	Forest sounds – People Animals Birds Wind Rain	Walking towards trees A forest Birds – which birds? Sing, song, tweet Under trees, dark, smell Grass, feels dry, feels wet Crunchy, crispy
Sit under a tree in a swing	Leaf chair Mosquito netting Leaves Fan Switch Bowl of dried leaves	Outdoor soundscape – Wind in leaves Crunch leaves Falling leaves	A swing Swinging in a swing Under a tree Falling leaves
Looking around the forest	Solar projector of leaves and people		Looking around Seeing trees, people
End of the day	Fibre-optic cave to look at the stars		Light fading Night falling I see stars

Susan Fowler and Helen Dilkes 2003

Copyright © Scope (Vic.) Ltd 2008

How to make your own projector wheels

(Subscribers feature article from ECAPPS newsletter, November 2001)

The easiest way to access the template for the projector wheel is to get somebody who already has a copy to e-mail it to you.

Otherwise, log onto the internet, get into ninemsn.com.au and do a web search, typing in 'projector wheels'. This will give you a list of websites to choose from.

Choose the site named 'How to make your own projector wheels'; once on this site, it will give you the option to download the template. It also states similar instructions as to the ones that follow but I have simplified it even more.

Open Microsoft Word and select File and save as a new document titled 'Projector Wheel Template.dot'.

A document like the one below should be visible. Now you are ready to import clip art and create your own projector wheel.

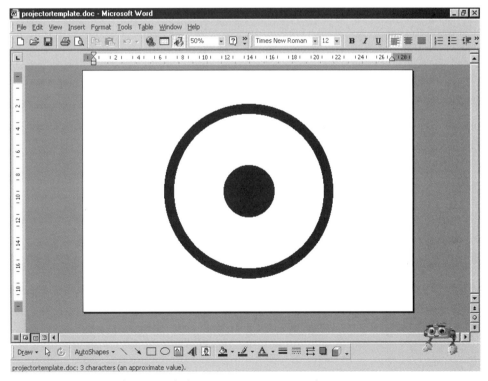

To start importing Clip Art, click Insert – Picture – Clip Art.

Copyright © Scope (Vic.) Ltd 2008

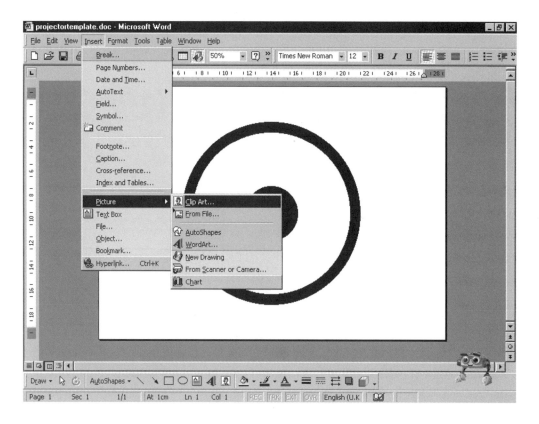

A window like the one below will appear. Scroll through the different themes until you find the images that you would like to use.

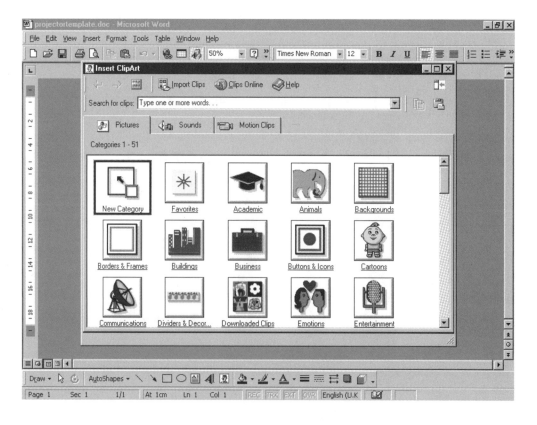

Double click on the chosen image and it will appear in your document below.

Copyright © Scope (Vic.) Ltd 2008

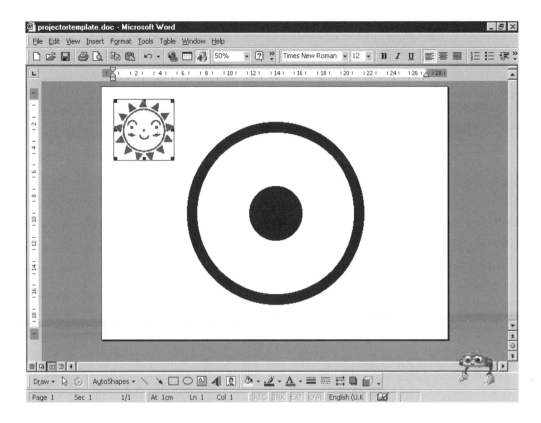

Click on a blank area of the page and repeat the process to add more Clip Art.

Now that you have imported all the images that you want we can start arranging them. First move the mouse over an image and click and drag to a blank area of the screen, but not in the large circle; repeat this for all of the images.

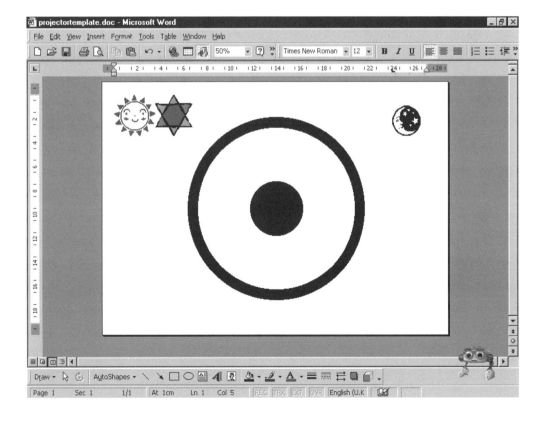

Some of the images may be too large or too small, but you can resize them if necessary; to do this, click on the image and nine boxes will appear around its perimeter. If you click on one of the corner boxes you can click and drag to change the size of the images.

Once all of the images have been resized to fit the wheel, click and drag them to move them to their rough places. In order to drag them you need to place each picture in front of the text. You need to do this to all pictures before placing them into the circle, otherwise they will not drag. To do this, click on the picture so that a box appears around it. Then click on Format on the tool bar and click on Picture. You will be given a series of tab headings. Click on Layout and then on the 'in front of text' icon. You will then be able to move your picture onto the wheel template.

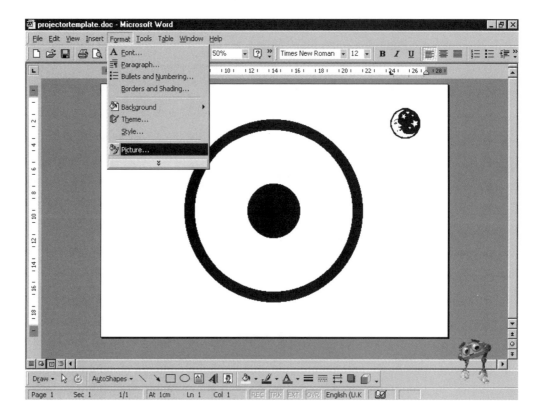

236   Copyright © Scope (Vic.) Ltd 2008

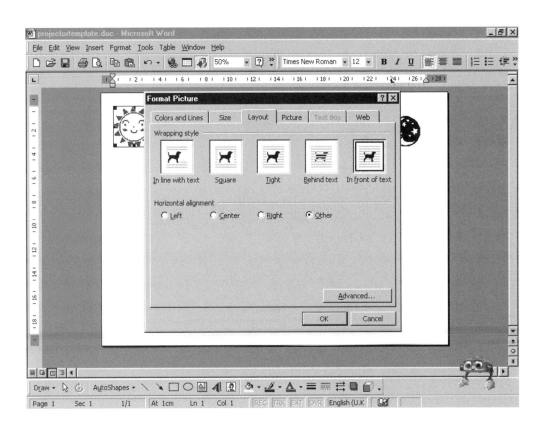

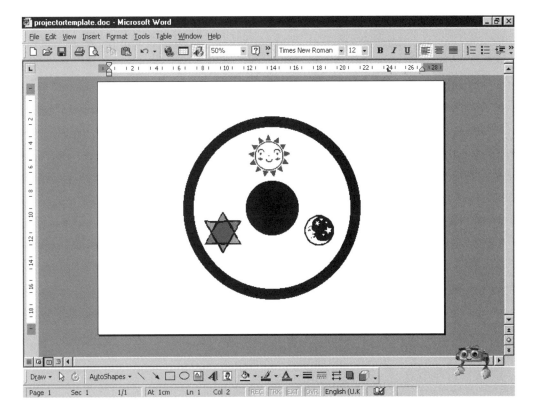

In order to rotate the pictures, we need some tools; to view the Drawing tools click on the icon on view, select Toolbars and then Drawing.

Copyright © Scope (Vic.) Ltd 2008

237

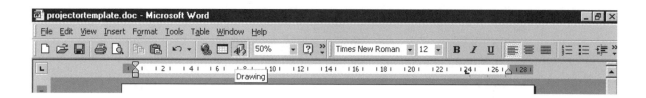

A toolbar like the one below will appear at the bottom of the screen.

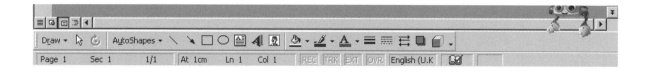

To rotate an image select the image by clicking on it, then click Draw – Ungroup.

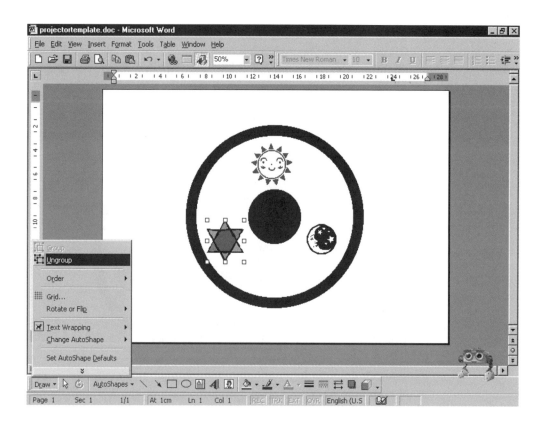

And then Draw – Group; this unlocks the image for editing.

 Copyright © Scope (Vic.) Ltd 2008

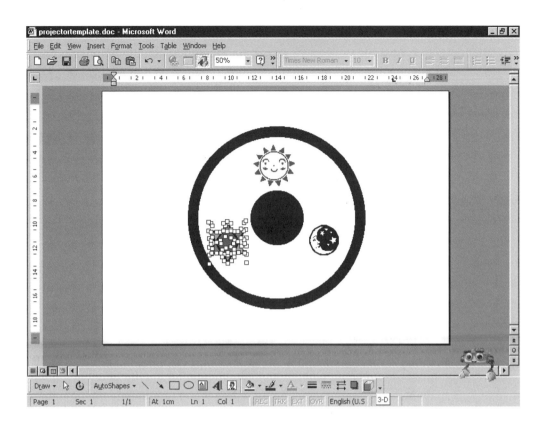

Now we click on the rotate icon. 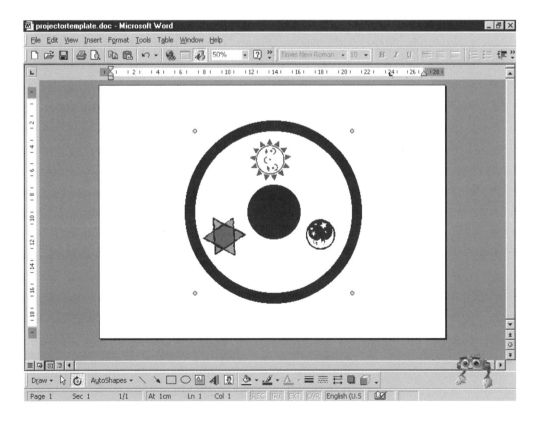 A green circle appears around the selected image and now we can start rotating. Click and Drag on one of the green circles to rotate the image to the correct position as shown below.

Next re-position any images that need it and save your file.

Copyright © Scope (Vic.) Ltd 2008

It is possible to add a fill colour or background to the wheel as an added effect. This is achieved by clicking on the wheel to select it and then clicking on the Fill icon (looks like a paint pot).

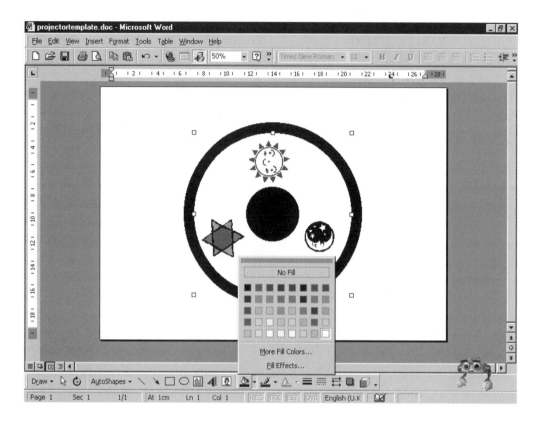

Click on the colour or click on Fill Effects to add an effect.

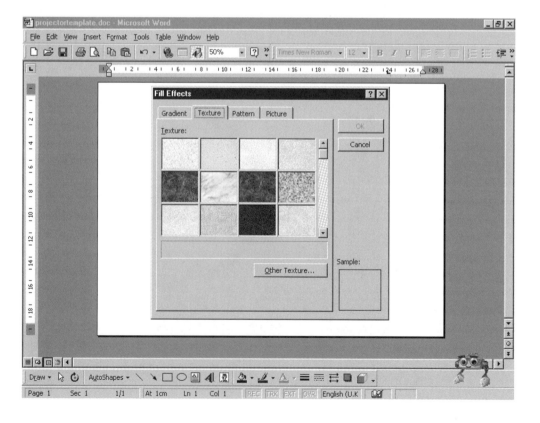

Copyright © Scope (Vic.) Ltd 2008

I clicked on the Texture tab and selected a bubble texture to go with the water theme. You could select a Gradient Fill, Pattern Fill or Picture. Click OK once you have made your choice. Your wheel will be updated with your chosen fill.

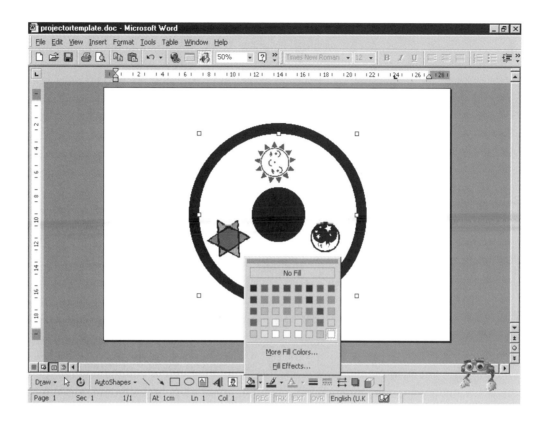

Projector wheels need to be printed on acetates. Make sure that you use an acetate recommended for use by your printer manufacturer; using incorrect or inferior acetates can make print quality suffer and void your printer warranty.

When printing projector wheels we print three sheets, allowing them to dry for several hours. We then overlay them using four drops of superglue in the centre of each sheet to hold them together. This ensures that we get a good depth of colour; using only one sheet creates a 'washed-out image'. To print on acetate select the correct setting in your printer software. If in doubt, consult the manual that came with your printer.

When the wheels have been cut out, insert them into blank wheels; these can be obtained from many multisensory equipment retailers. Finally, attach the wheel to a rpm rotator, insert into a projector and enjoy your new wheel.

Discovery room activities

The following are activities designed by Suzanne Rizzo, a teacher at Nepean Special School, Melbourne, Australia, where the multisensory room (called the discovery room) has been used for Maths, English and health/PE activities.

English		
Activity	**What to do**	**Equipment**
Speech Vocalization Singing	Encourage use of the microphone Play some of the student's favourite songs on the sound system to encourage vocalization, singing and speech	Microphone (water bed, infinity tunnel and coloured light ladder) Echo tube Sound system
Shared reading Reading activities Literature	Set the scene; the choice is yours – e.g. story about water or marine life – bubble column and deep sea projected image on the wall	Quiet room
Colours	Find the same colour	Quiet room Catherine wheel Activity board UV light
Specific colour	Press the red (or whatever colour you decide) button and turn off the catherine wheel (blu tac a round red circle the same size as the button on the catherine wheel)	Catherine wheel
Choice making	Use a pictograph that has been made and displayed on activity room wall	Quiet room or activity room and the choices within these rooms

Copyright © Scope (Vic.) Ltd 2008

Following instructions	E.g. hide a favourite toy and give clues: 'It is near the bubbles'; this activity can be as simple or as complex as you need it to be	Quiet room Activity room
Role play Dressing up	Imagine if…	Quiet room Activity room UV section

Maths		
Activity	**What to do**	**Equipment**
Shapes and patterns	Use UV long cords and make shapes and patterns: □ △ ○ Use fluoro shoe laces and glue into shapes and patterns on black paper	UV light
Develop concepts – up/down in/out on/off high/low	E.g. activity board Up/down or both – light ladder, ball chute, light chaser In/out or both – ball chute, lucky dip bag, echo tube On/off or both – musical panel, vibrating panel, cow, cat, light chaser High/low or both – light ladder, reach high to press the musical panel and get down low to press the cow or cat	Quiet room Activity room

Copyright © Scope (Vic.) Ltd 2008

Health and PE

Activity	What to do	Equipment
Relaxation	Lie in favourite part of the quiet room	Quiet room equipment Soft playing music Dimmed coloured lights
Leisure	Free choice of quiet or activity room for independent play	Use all equipment in quiet and activity rooms
Physiotherapy	Standing in frames or out on mats, wedges or rollers Students are positioned in front of favourite equipment in quiet or activity rooms	Use all equipment in quiet and activity rooms
Gross motor	Walking, crawling and stretched out on musical mat	Musical mat
Massage	Use a hand cream or an oil you may have been using in your room for massage programmes	All equipment in the quiet room Hand cream Aromatherapy oil
Footspa	Use an oil you may have been using in your room for massage programmes or match it with the oil in the aromatherapy	All equipment in the quiet room Foot spa Aromatherapy oil
Bubble blowing	Adult can blow bubbles in the air to observe Students can blow bubbles	All equipment in the quiet room Bubble equipment
Parachute	All go under the parachute – What can you hear? (music, bubble column) What can you see? (mirror ball lights)	Quiet room

Copyright © Scope (Vic.) Ltd 2008

Glossary

Activity Arch

A metal or plastic frame that is set up over a wheelchair or someone lying/sitting on the floor. Different sensory objects are suspended from the frame so that a person can reach out and explore the different objects

Bubble Tube

Perspex tubes containing water and mounted to a base which contains a pump, light and colour wheel. The pump creates tiny bubbles which float up the clear perspex tube and as the colour wheel rotates, it seems to make the bubbles change colour.

Co-active assistance

A method of assisting people to participate in an activity or explore an object. The support person moves the other person's body part (e.g. arm) so that they can experience the movement associated with operating equipment or exploring an object. One method of co-active assistance is when the support person supports the other person's hand and elbow. In this way, the support person can assist the other to reach forward to press a switch, feel an object or use an object functionally (e.g. pour milk from a jug).

Complex communication

Having little or no speech

Complex Communication Needs: "People with Complex Communication Needs have communication problems associated with a wide range of physical, sensory and environmental causes which restrict/limit their ability to participate independently in society. They and their communication partners may benefit from using augmentative and alternative communication (AAC) methods either temporarily or permanently" (Balandin,2002).

Designed Multisensory Environment

Any environment that's designed to provide multisensory experiences. This includes rooms, gardens, activity arches, verandas and ramps

Fibre Optic Spray

A series of thin glass or plastic fibres of varying length used with a light source. The glass fibres are encased in plastic and transmit different coloured lights as the colour wheel rotates in front of the light source.

Intensive interaction

Intensive interaction describes a way of communicating with people with profound and multiple disabilities. It is based on the interaction style that a parent has with a young baby and the focus is on the process of interaction rather than it's outcome.

Interactive cushions

These are full seats (base and back) or backrest only, which can be connected to computers, DVD's and CD players. This enables people to hear and feel the vibrations from music and games.

Leaf chair

A soft padded seat that cradles the body and is suspended from the ceiling or standing frame. The seat provides support and as it is suspended provides a gentle bouncing or swinging motion

Mirror Ball

Ball covered with mirror tiles and mounted with a motor so that the mirror balls can rotate. They vary in size and can be suspended from the ceiling or small battery operated ones can be mounted on a stand. They are often used with a light and colour wheel so that different colours can be projected onto the mirror ball. This produces different coloured spots of light that move around the room when the mirror ball is rotated.

Multisensory Room

A specific room that is designed to provide multisensory experiences. The difference between a "snoezelen" room and a multisensory room is how the room is used. The emphasis in a "snoezelen" room is on relaxation and leisure, whilst a multisensory room is also used for therapeutic and educational needs.

Object engagement

Any behaviour where the person engages with an object in a purposeful way e.g. looking at, tracking, reaching for, holding and using the object in a functional way.

Object Symbol

An object or partial object used to represent an activity. This is used as a cue to alert people to an activity that is about to occur.

Personal Communication Dictionary

Is used with people who are unintentional communicators and is a way of recording an individual's way of communicating. It is presented as a table documenting what a person does, what you think it means and how you should respond.

Person engagement

Any behaviours where the person engages with another person e.g. making eye contact, watching a person moving around the room, reaching to a person, vocalising at and smiling at another person.

Person-Object engagement

Any behaviour where the person engages with an object and person at the same time e.g. looking at a person and an object (shared attention), giving an object to a person.

Power box

A piece of equipment used to make any electrical appliance switch accessible. External switches are plugged into the power box which allows people to turn on appliances without needing good fine motor skills.

Self-engagement behaviour

Any repetitive behaviours where a person engages with their body or their clothing. Self engagement behaviours which include rocking & finger flicking can be self-stimulating or they may be used to calm a person in an overstimulating environment.

Sensory Banks

Collections of different types of materials and equipment, categorised according to the different senses. Some sensory banks may be categorised into themes e.g. sensory items for the garden or beach.

Sensory profile

A way of describing each persons unique sensory needs For example, some people may be easily over stimulated and others may need more stimulation to take notice of the things around them.

The Sensory Profile (Dunn 1999) is also an evaluation tool which poses a number of questions in relation to behavioural responses to everyday sensory experiences.

Shared attention

Part of person-object engagement behaviour, where people alternate their gaze between a person and an object. Both people therefore attend to the same object or event. The individual is sharing an activity with another person.

Snoezelen

The Snoezelen approach focuses on enjoying environments that stimulate the senses, without trying to analyse those experiences.

Snoezelen Rooms have been developed where the emphasis is on providing multisensory experiences within a specific room. However, Snoezelen can occur in any environment where the emphasis is on using the senses.

Solar Effects Projector

A light unit that is used with cassettes or wheels to project images onto different surfaces, such as walls, ceilings, white umbrella's & white lycra screens

Soundbeam

A piece of equipment comprising an ultrasonic sensor & control box. The soundbeam needs to be connected to a midi keyboard or sound module as these produce the sounds. This creates an invisible keyboard or musical instrument in space that can be "played" through peoples' movements in front of the sensor. The length and width of space where people can operate the soundbeam is variable so that people can blink an eye or dance around to trigger soundbeam.

Soundbox

A hollow box containing speakers. People sit or lie on the box so that they can feel the music resonating through the box.

Tactile wall

Wall panel made from various textures that can be obtained commercially or made. The wall panels can be freestanding but often are secured to walls. They are frequently divided into sections with different textures in the different sections. Some walls also contain vibrating panels and items which stimulate other senses e.g. musical instruments, smell tubes, light displays

Unintentional communication

A level of communication where support people allocate meaning to a person's behaviour.

UV objects

Objects that glow when looked at under UV (ultra violet) light. UV is part of the spectrum of light that is at the violet end.

Vibroacoustic beanbags/body pillow

Beanbags & pillows containing speakers. The beanbags or pillows are linked to a sound system so that people can feel the vibrations from the music (the base notes provide more intense input) as well as listen to the music.

Vibroacoustic bed

A bed that contain speakers and is linked to a sound system. People can lie or sit on the bed and feel the vibrations from the music

Vibrating bed

A bed containing an element that vibrates so that a person can sit or lie on the bed and be massaged by the vibrations.

References

Ashby, M., Lindsay, W., Pitcaithly, D., Broxholme, S. and Geelen, N. (1995) 'Snoezelen: Its effects on concentration and responsiveness in people with profound multiple handicaps.' *British Journal of Occupational Therapy 58*, 7, 303–307.

Ayres, M. (2001) *Sensory Resources Catalogue No. 1*. Available at: www.mikeayresdesign.co.uk, accessed June 2008.

Baker, R., Dowling, Z., Wareing, L.A., Dawson, J. and Assey, J. (1997) 'Snoezelen: Its long-term and short-term effects on older people with dementia.' *British Journal of Occupational Therapy 60*, 5, 213–218.

Brinker, R.P. and Lewis, M. (1982) 'Making the world work with microcomputers: A learning prosthesis for handicapped infants.' *Exceptional Children 49*, 2, 163–170.

Burns, I., Cox, H. and Plant, H. (2000) 'Leisure or therapeutics? Snoezelen and the care of older persons with dementia.' *International Journal of Nursing Practice 6*, 118–126.

Cuvo, A.J., May, M.E. and Post, T.M. (2001) 'Effects of living room, Snoezelen room, and outdoor activities on stereotypic behaviour and engagement by adults with profound metal retardation.' *Research in Developmental Disabilities 22*, 183–204.

de Bunsen, A. (1994) 'A Study in the Implication of the Snoezelen Resources at Limington House School.' In R. Hutchinson and J. Kewin (eds) *Sensations and Disability: Sensory Environments for Leisure, Snoezelen, Education and Therapy*. Chesterfield: ROMPA.

Don, M. (2001) *The Sensuous Garden*. London: Conran Octopus.

Glenn, S., Cunningham, C. and Shorrock, A. (1996) 'Social Interaction in Multi-Sensory Environments.' In N. Bozic and H. Murdock (eds) *Learning through Interaction: Technology and Children with Multiple Disabilities*. London: David Fulton Publishers.

Hagger, E. and Hutchinson, R. (1991) 'Snoezelen: An approach to the provision of a leisure resource for people with profound and multiple handicaps.' *Mental Handicap 19*, 51–55.

Hirstwood, R. and Grey, M. (1995) *A Practical Guide to the Use of Multisensory Rooms*. Leicestershire: TFH.

Hogg, J., Cavet, J., Lambe, L. and Smeddle, M. (2001) 'The use of "Snoezelen" as multisensory stimulation with people with intellectual disabilities: A review of the research.' *Research in Developmental Disabilities 22*, 353–372.

Hope, K. (1997) 'Using multi-sensory environments with older people with dementia.' *Journal of Advanced Nursing 25*, 4, 780–785.

Horticultural Therapy Association of Victoria (1996) *An Introduction to Raised Garden Beds*. Victoria: Embassy Press.

Horticultural Therapy Association of Victoria (1997) *Sensory Gardens for Horticultural Therapy Programs*. Victoria: Embassy Press.

Houghton, S., Douglas, G., Brigg, J., Langsford, S., Powell, L., West, J., Chapman, A. and Kellner, R. (1998) 'An empirical evaluation of an interactive multi-sensory environment for children with disability.' *Journal of Intellectual and Developmental Disability 23*, 4, 267–278.

Hulsegge, J. and Verheul, A. (1987) *Snoezelen: Another World*. Chesterfield: ROMPA.

Hutchinson, R. and Haggar, L. (1994) 'The Development and Evaluation of a Snoezelen Leisure Resource for People with Severe Multiple Disabilities.' In R. Hutchinson and J. Kewin (eds)

Sensations and Disability: Sensory Environments for Leisure, Snoezelen, Education and Therapy. Chesterfield: ROMPA.

Hutchinson, R. and Kewin, J. (1994) *Sensations and Disability.* Chesterfield: ROMPA.

Jamieson, P. (1995) *The Music Man* (song is 'Silver Balloon'). CD. Available at: www.themusicman.com.au, accessed February 2008.

Jones, G. and Crawford, H. (2005) 'Making sense of the classroom.' *Special Children,* July/August, 37–38.

Kenyon, J. and Hong, C.S. (1998) 'An explorative study of the function of a multisensory environment.' *British Journal of Therapy and Rehabilitation 5,* 12, 619–623.

Lindsay, W.R., Pitcaithly, D., Geelen, N., Buntin, L., Broxholme, S. and Ashby, M. (1997) 'A comparison of the effects of four therapy procedures on concentration and responsiveness in people with profound learning disabilities.' *Journal of Intellectual Disability Research 41,* 3, 201–207.

Long, A. and Haig, L. (1992) 'How do clients benefit from Snoezelen? An exploratory study.' *British Journal of Occupational Therapy 55,* 3, 103–106..

Longhorn, F. (1988) *A Sensory Curriculum for Very Special People: A Practical Approach to Curriculum Planning.* London: Souvenir Press.

Longhorn, F. (1997) *Enhancing Education through the Use of Ultraviolet Light and Fluorescing Materials.* Bedfordshire: Catalyst Education Resources Limited.

Longhorn, F. (2001) *Sensory Drama for Very Special People.* Bedfordshire: Catalyst Education Resources Limited.

Martin, N., Gaffan, R. and Williams, T. (1998) 'Behavioural effects of long-term multi-sensory stimulation.' *British Journal of Clinical Psychology 37,* 69–83.

McKenzie, C. (1995) 'Brightening the lives of elderly residents through Snoezelen.' *Elderly Care 7,* 5, 11–13.

McLarty, M. (1993) 'Soap opera or bubble tube?' *Eye Contact,* Autumn, 11–12.

Moffat, N., Barker, P., Pinkney, L., Garside, M. and Freeman, C. (1993) *Snoezelen: An Experience for People with Dementia.* Chesterfield: ROMPA.

Morrissey, M. (1997) 'Snoezelen: Benefits for nursing older clients.' *Nursing Standard 12,* 3, 38–40.

Mount, H. and Cavet, J. (1995) 'Multi-sensory environments: An exploration of their potential for young people with profound and multiple learning difficulties.' *British Journal of Special Education 22,* 2, 52–55..

Nind, M. and Hewitt, D. (2001) *A Practical Guide to Intensive Interaction.* Kidderminster: BILD Publications.

O'Brien, J. (1989) *What's Worth Working For? Leadership for Better Quality Human Services.* Georgia, USA: Responsive Systems Associates.

O'Brien, Y., Glen, S.M., and Cunningham, C.C. (1994) 'Contingency awareness in infants and children with severe and profound learning disabilities.' *International Journal of Disability. Development and Education 41,* 231–243.

Orr, R. (1993) 'Life beyond the room?' *Eye Contact 6,* 25–26.

Pagliano, P. (1999) *Multisensory Environments.* London: David Fulton Publishers.

Pagliano, P. (2001) *Using a Multisensory Environment: A Practical Guide for Teachers.* London: David Fulton Publishers.

Pinkney, L. and Barker, P. (1994) 'Snoezelen: An Evaluation of a Sensory Environment Used by People who are Elderly and Confused.' In R. Hutchinson and J. Kewin (eds) *Sensations and Disability: Sensory Environments for Leisure, Snoezelen, Education and Therapy.* Chesterfield: ROMPA.

REFERENCES

Sanderson, H. and Harrison, J. (1996) *Aromatherapy and Massage for People with Learning Difficulties.* London: Hands on Publishing.

Schofield, P. (1996) 'Snoezelen: Its potential for people with chronic pain.' *Complementary Therapies in Nursing and Midwifery 2*, 9–12.

Schofield, P. (2000) 'The effects of Snoezelen on chronic pain.' *Nursing Standard 15*, 1, 33–34.

Schofield, P. and Davies, B. (1998) 'Sensory deprivation and chronic pain: A review of the literature.' *Disability and Rehabilitation 20*, 20, 357–366.

Schofield, P., Davies, B. and Hutchinson, R. (1998) 'Snoezelen and chronic pain: Developing a study to evaluate its use (Part I).' *Complementary Therapies in Nursing and Midwifery 4*, 66–72.

Shapiro, M., Parush, S., Green, M. and Roth, D. (1997) 'The efficacy of the "Snoezelen" in the management of children with mental retardation who exhibit maladaptive behaviours.' *British Journal of Developmental Disabilities 43*, 85, 140–155.

Slevin, E. and McClelland, A. (1999) 'Multisensory environments: Are they therapeutic? A single-subject evaluation of the clinical effectiveness of a multisensory environment.' *Journal of Clinical Nursing 8*, 1, 48–56.

Terry, P. and Hong, C.S. (1998) 'People with learning disabilities and multisensory environments.' *British Journal of Therapy and Rehabilitation 5*, 12, 630–633.

Thompson, S.B.N. and Martin, S. (1994) 'Making sense of multisensory rooms for people with learning disabilities.' *British Journal of Occupational Therapy 57*, 341–344.

Vlaskamp, C., Geeter, K., Liselot, M. and Smit, I. (2003) 'Passive activities: The effectiveness of multisensory environments on the level of activity of individuals with profound multiple disabilities.' *Journal of Applied Research in Intellectual Disabilities 16*, 135–143.

White, J. (1997) 'Creating a Snoezelen effect in PICU.' *Paediatric Nursing 9*, 5, 20–21.

Whittaker, J. (1992) 'Can anyone help me to understand the logic of Snoezelen? Asks Joe Whittaker.' *Community Living*, October, 15.

Wilcox, S. (1994) 'Snoezelen in elderly care.' *British Journal of Occupational Therapy 57*, 6, 242.

Woodrow, P. (1998) 'Interventions for confusion and dementia 4: Alternative approaches.' *British Journal of Nursing 7*, 20, 1247–1250.